Textbook of
Operation Theatre
Technology

Textbook of
Operation Theatre
Technology

Manjushree Ray

MBBS, MD (Anaesthesiology), MAMS, FICA

Principal
Medical College,
Kolkata, West Bengal

MM Ray MBBS, MS (Orthopaedics)

Former Professor and Head
Department of Orthopaedics
Medical College, Kolkata

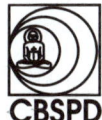

CBSPD

CBS Publishers & Distributors Pvt Ltd

New Delhi • Bengaluru • Chennai • Kochi • Kolkata • Lucknow • Mumbai
Hyderabad • Jharkhand • Nagpur • Patna • Pune • Uttarakhand

Textbook of
Operation Theatre
Technology

ISBN: 978-93-89396-21-8

Copyright © Authors and Publisher

First Edition: 2020

Reprint: 2022, 2024

Published by Satish Kumar Jain and produced by Varun Jain for

CBS Publishers & Distributors Pvt Ltd

4819/XI Prahlad Street, 24 Ansari Road, Daryaganj, New Delhi 110 002, India
Ph: 011-23289259, 23266861   Website: www.cbspd.com
                                     e-mail: delhi@cbspd.com

Corporate Office: 204 FIE, Industrial Area, Patparganj, Delhi 110 092
Ph: 011-4934 4934   Fax: 011-4934 4935   e-mail: publishing@cbspd.com; publicity@cbspd.com

Branches

- **Bengaluru:** Seema House 2975, 17th Cross, K.R. Road, Banasankari 2nd Stage, Bengaluru 560 070, Karnataka, India
  Ph: +91-80-26771678/79   Fax: +91-80-26771680   e-mail: bangalore@cbspd.com
- **Chennai:** 7, Subbaraya Street, Shenoy Nagar, Chennai 600 030, Tamil Nadu, India
  Ph: +91-44-26680620, 26681266   Fax: +91-44-42032115   e-mail: chennai@cbspd.com
- **Kochi:** 42/1325, 1326, Power House Road, Opp KSEB, Power House, Ernakulam Kochi 682 018, Kerala, India
  Ph: +91-484-4059061-65, 67   Fax: +91-484-4059065   e-mail: kochi@cbspd.com
- **Kolkata:** 147, Hind Ceramics Compound, 1st Floor, Nilgunj Road, Belghoria, Kolkata-700056, West Bengal, India
  Ph: 033-25633055, 033-25633056   e-mail: kolkata@cbspd.com
- **Lucknow:** Basement, Khushnuma Complex, 7-Meerabai Marg (Behind Jawahar Bhawan), Lucknow 226001, UP, India
  Ph: 0522-4000032   e-mail: tiwari.lucknow@cbspd.com
- **Mumbai:** PWD Shed. Gala no. 25/26, Ramchandra Bhatt Marg, Next to JJ Hospital Gate no. 2, Opp. Union Bank of India, Noorbaug, Mumbai-400009, Maharashtra, India
  Ph: 022-66661880/89   e-mail: mumbai@cbspd.com

Representatives

- **Hyderabad** 0-9885175004   • **Jharkhand** 0-9811541605   • **Nagpur**   0-9421945513
- **Patna**   0-9334159340   • **Pune**   0-9923910676   • **Uttarakhand** 0-9716462459

Printed at Goyal Offset Works Pvt. Ltd., Kundli, Haryana, India

Foreword

"Making the simple complicated is commonplace; making the complicated simple, awesomely simple, that's creativity"
— *Charles Mingus*

When the operation theatre technology course was initiated, obviously there was requirement for course material. There was no available book in the market which can deal with the requirement of the students of operation theatre technology. At that time, author took up the responsibility to develop such material, as this course was just like a brainchild for her. I requested her to make it not only simple and lucid for the students, but also to ignite their interest for the subject.

"We really are living in an age of information overload. Google has estimated that there are 300 exabytes (300 followed by 18 zeros) of human made information in the world today. Only four years ago, there were just 30 exabytes. We have created more information in the past few years than in all of human history before us."
— *Daniel Levitin*

This makes us inattentive about the real need of the students and we try to overburden them.

"A wealth of information creates a poverty of attention."
— *Herbert Simon*

The author not only has kept my request, but also thought for the teachers and examiners. Majority of us, faculties tend to forget, who are the targeted learners and quite often overshoot the boundaries. The author has also taken all these in consideration and this book can really function as a framed guideline for the faculties also.

I personally pray to Almighty to bless the authors and their creation.

Debasis Bhattacharyya
Director of Medical Education
Department of Health and Family Welfare, West Bengal

Preface

The twentieth century witnessed tremendous advancement in the field of medicine, that too in operation theatre technology. Needless to say that the technologists in operation theatre (OT) have to handle medical instruments and equipment for the surgical procedures of the patients. Therefore, they need to have updated knowledge in OT technology and human biology. The book is written with an eye to impart optimum knowledge required for the technologists.

It has 52 chapters which cover the entire syllabus of operation theatre course for the technologists. It includes basic science covering human anatomy, physiology and biochemistry of all systems. This knowledge of human biology will help the learners to grasp the clinical procedures performed in the theatre. Besides, they are expected to have enough knowledge of OT structure and functioning that has been laid out here in detail. Sterilization of instruments and maintenance thereof are also important issues in any surgical procedure which has been aptly explained in related chapters. The learners will also be able to know the care of pre- and postoperative patients in the OT complex. The technique of handling patients and their transport has been detailed in the book.

Technologists will be benefitted with the knowledge of common surgical conditions of the patients depicted in section IV here. At the same time, routine surgical procedures have duly been explained to enable the OT technologists to assist surgeon efficiently. They have a major role in helping anaesthesiologist and maintaining anaesthesia machine. They too should know the anaesthetic drugs and their uses. This part has been highlighted with the importance it deserves. The maintenance of instruments and equipment has been described for the technologists to do their job systematically and scientifically. Special surgical and diagnostic procedures like endoscopic surgery and diagnostic endoscopy have been included in the book with a view to enabling them to work in superspeciality hospitals.

As the technologists are dealing with the patients and deeply involved with their treatment, they must have enough knowledge of medical ethics, and communication skill as well. This aspect too has been written in a comprehensive manner. The language used here is very simple and easy to follow.

We sincerely hope that this book will be a unique practical source of information to the learners of operation theater technology.

Manjushree Ray
MM Ray

Contents

SECTION V: ANAESTHESIA AND COMMON PERIOPERATIVE COMPLICATIONS

SECTION VI: COMMON EQUIPMENT OF OPERATION THEATRE: CLEANING AND MAINTENANCE

SECTION VII: TECHNIQUES OF COMMON CLINICAL PROCEDURES

SECTION VIII: ETHICS AND COMMUNICATIONS

CHAPTER **1**

Introduction to Anatomy and Physiology of Human Body

The human body can be considered as a highly technical and sophisticated machine that operates as a single unit consisting of a number of systems, which work independently.

Anatomy and physiology are the branches of medical science, deal with structures and functions of the different parts of the body, respectively.

STRUCTURAL ORGANIZATION OF THE HUMAN BODY

Atom

The most fundamental structure of a human body is chemical and atom is the smallest part of it. Examples: Carbon, hydrogen and oxygen atoms.

Molecules and Macromolecules

- Atoms combine to form molecules such as H_2O and CO_2. Molecules combine and form macromolecules such as carbohydrates, lipids and proteins.
- Various combinations of these macromolecules develop nucleus, mitochondria, ribosomes, golgi apparatus, etc. Each of them plays a very important and specific role within a cell.

Cells

- They are the smallest independent units of the human body. There are different types of cells depending upon the specialized job performed by them.
- Different types of cells can be distinguished microscopically by their shapes, sizes and dye they absorb on staining at the laboratory.

Tissues

Cells with similar structures and functions are found together and form tissues. Examples: Connective tissue, epithelial tissue, muscular tissue and nervous tissue.

Organs

They are made of different types of tissues and are assigned to carry out a specific function. Examples: Stomach, brain and heart.

Systems

System consists of a number of organs contribute together to carry out one or more survival needs of the body (Table 1.1).

BODY CAVITIES

Body cavities contain and protect different vital organs of the body. There are four body

Table 1.1	Activities of different systems
Survival need	Activities of systems
Communication	Nervous system Endocrine system
Transport	Cardiovascular system Blood
Intake of raw materials and elimination of waste products	Gastrointestinal system Respiratory system Excretory system
Protection and survivals	Skin Musculoskeletal system Reproductive system

cavities—cranial cavity, thoracic cavity, abdominal cavity and pelvic cavity.

Cranial Cavity

- The cranial cavity is consisting of bones of the skull which protects brain.

Boundaries

- Anteriorly—1 frontal bone
- Laterally—2 temporal bones
- Posteriorly—1 occipital bone
- Superiorly—2 parietal bones
- Inferiorly—1 sphenoid and 1 ethmoid bone

Thoracic Cavity

Thoracic cavity is situated in the upper part of the trunk. It contains following organs.
- A part of the gastrointestinal system— oesophagus
- Part of the respiratory system—trachea, bronchi and lungs
- Part of the cardiovascular system—heart, aorta, superior and inferior vena cava and other major blood vessels.

Boundaries

- Anteriorly—sternum and costal cartilage of ribs
- Laterally—twelve pairs of ribs and inter- costal muscles

- Posteriorly—thoracic vertebrae
- Superiorly—structures forming the root of the neck
- Inferiorly—diaphragm muscle

Abdominal Cavity

It is located in the middle part of the trunk. It contains following organs.
- Most of the gastrointestinal system— stomach, small and large intestine, liver, gallbladder, bile ducts and pancreas
- Part of the excretory system—two kidneys and ureters
- Other organs—spleen, lymph nodes and adrenal glands

Boundaries

- Superiorly—diaphragm muscle
- Anteriorly—muscles forming anterior abdominal wall
- Posteriorly—lumbar vertebrae and muscles forming posterior abdominal wall
- Laterally—lower ribs and muscles of the abdominal wall
- Inferiorly—continues with the pelvic cavity.

Regions of Abdominal Cavity

For a better understanding of the position of structures, the abdominal cavity is divided into 9 regions by two vertical and two horizontal lines (Fig. 1.1).
- Right hypochondriac region
- Epigastric region
- Left hypochondriac region
- Right lumbar region
- Umbilical region
- Left lumbar region
- Right iliac fossa
- Hypogastric region
- Left iliac fossa

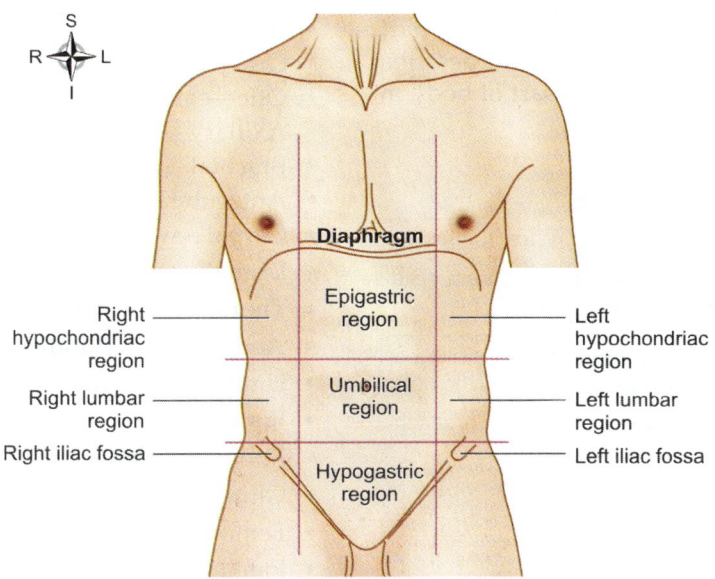

Fig. 1.1: Abdominal regions

Anatomical Terminology (Fig. 1.2)

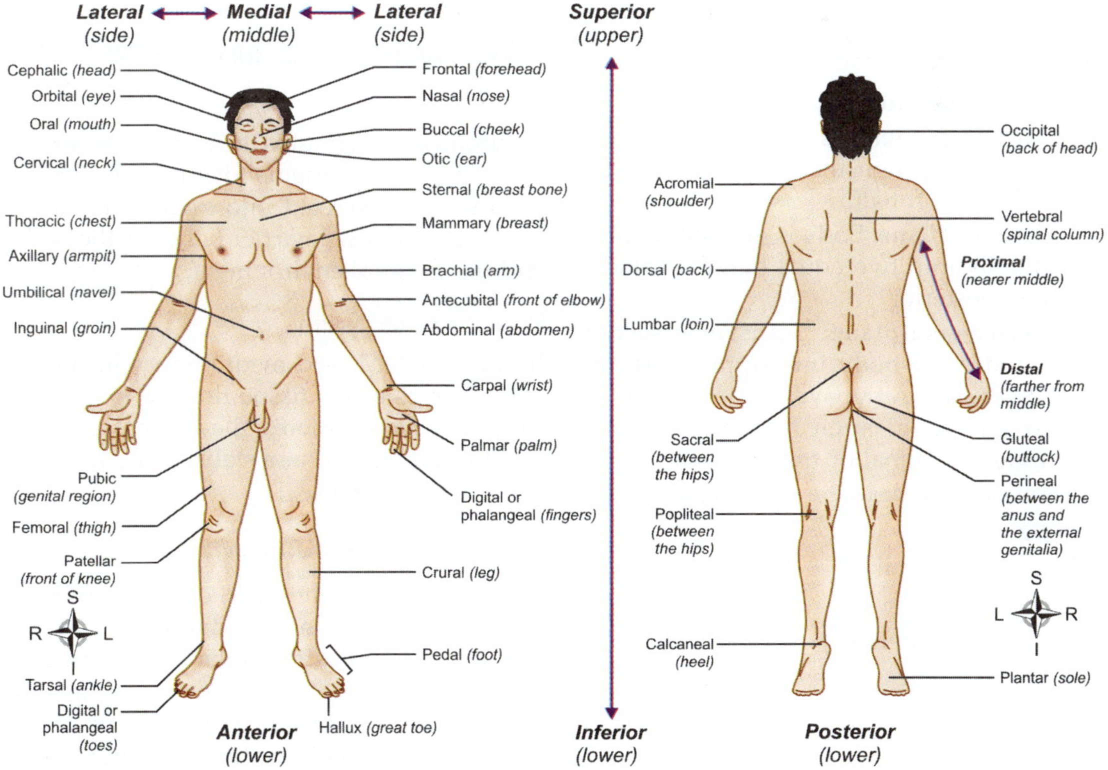

Lateral ⟷ **Medial** ⟷ **Lateral**   **Superior**
(side)   *(middle)*   *(side)*   *(upper)*

Cephalic *(head)*
Orbital *(eye)*
Oral *(mouth)*
Cervical *(neck)*
Thoracic *(chest)*
Axillary *(armpit)*
Umbilical *(navel)*
Inguinal *(groin)*
Pubic *(genital region)*
Femoral *(thigh)*
Patellar *(front of knee)*
Tarsal *(ankle)*
Digital or phalangeal *(toes)*

Frontal *(forehead)*
Nasal *(nose)*
Buccal *(cheek)*
Otic *(ear)*
Sternal *(breast bone)*
Mammary *(breast)*
Brachial *(arm)*
Antecubital *(front of elbow)*
Abdominal *(abdomen)*
Carpal *(wrist)*
Palmar *(palm)*
Digital or phalangeal *(fingers)*
Crural *(leg)*
Pedal *(foot)*
Hallux *(great toe)*

Anterior *(lower)*

Acromial *(shoulder)*
Dorsal *(back)*
Lumbar *(loin)*
Sacral *(between the hips)*
Popliteal *(between the hips)*
Calcaneal *(heel)*

Occipital *(back of head)*
Vertebral *(spinal column)*
Proximal *(nearer middle)*
Distal *(farther from middle)*
Gluteal *(buttock)*
Perineal *(between the anus and the external genitalia)*
Plantar *(sole)*

Inferior *(lower)*   **Posterior** *(lower)*

Fig. 1.2: Body regions (anatomical terminology)

1. **Terms related to relative position of a part of body:** Different terms used to describe the position of a particular part of body in relations to other parts:

Term	Meaning
Superior	Above or nearer to head
Inferior	Below or farther from head
Medial	Nearer to midline
Lateral	Farther from the midline or towards the side of the body
Proximal	Nearer to the point of attachment of a limb
Distal	Farther from the point of attachment of a limb
Anterior or ventral	Nearer to the front of the body
Posterior or dorsal	Nearer to the back of the body
Cephaloid or cephalic	Nearer to head
Caudal	Nearer to tail

2. **Terms related to body planes:**
   - **Median plane:** Body is divided longitudinally through the midline into right half and left half.
   - **Coronal plane:** Body is divided longitudinally into two equal halves anterior and posterior
   - **Transverse plane:** Transverse section divides the body into upper part and lower part. A transverse section may be at any level such as transthoracic, transabdominal or transcranial.

3. **Terms used to describe various parts of the body:**
   - Cranial—skull
   - Nasal—nose
   - Frontal—forehead
   - Orbital—eye
   - Facial—face
   - Cervical—neck
   - Cephalic—head

- Buccal—cheek
- Oral—mouth
- Otic—ear
- Axillary—armpit
- Brachial—upper arm
- Antecubital—anterior elbow
- Carpal—wrist
- Digital—finger
- Thoracic—chest
- Abdominal—abdomen
- Umbilical—navel
- Inguinal—groin
- Pubic—genital region
- Gluteal—buttocks
- Femoral—thigh
- Patellar—front of knee
- Tarsal—ankle
- Popliteal—back of the knee
- Plantar—sole

ENVIRONMENT OF THE HUMAN BODY

External Environment

Environment surrounds the body is the source of oxygen and nutrients for the body. Waste products are excreted into external environment. The skin is a barrier between the body and the external environment.

Internal Environment

It is the water-based medium in which cells exist. This is called tissue fluid or interstitial fluid. The composition of the internal environment is maintained at a stable state, which is called homeostasis.

BODY FLUID COMPARTMENTS

Body fluid constitutes 60% of the total body weight. They are mainly distributed in the intracellular and extracellular compartments.

- **Extracellular fluid:** Water present outside the cells is extracellular fluid. It is about one-third of total body fluid distributed into interstitial space and plasma.

- **Intracellular fluid:** It constitutes about two-thirds of total body fluids and presents within the cells.
- **Others:** CSF, GI secretions, serous fluids

Water Balance

- Total water intake by an adult—2500 ml/day
  - Source:
    - Water ingestion—60%
    - Intake through food—30%
    - Cell metabolism—10%
- Total output of water—2500 ml/day
    - Urine from the kidney—60%
    - Evaporation through the skin—28%
    - Perspiration—8%
    - Faeces—4%

Electrolyte Balance

Concentrations of electrolytes within body fairly remains constant. Serum sodium, potassium, calcium, magnesium and chloride levels are maintained within normal range by various mechanisms.

- Sodium balance is maintained by aldo-sterone, antidiuretic hormone and atrial natriuretic factors.

- Potassium level is regulated at kidney mainly by aldosterone.
- Calcium is mostly absorbed in bones and this is regulated by two hormones—parathyroid and calcitonin.

Acid–Base Balance

- Normally pH of the fluid is maintained between 7.34 and 7.43.
- Body acid–base balance is basically maintained by the respiratory and excretory systems.

COMMON TERMINOLOGY ASSOCIATED WITH THE DISEASE

Aetiology: Cause of disease

Pathogenesis: The main process causing disease

Complications: Consequence which may occur with the progress of the disease

Prognosis: Likely outcome

Acute: Sudden onset of disease

Chronic: Long-standing disorder

Congenital: Disorder presents since birth

Acquired: Disorder develops after birth

Communicable: Disease spread from one person to other.

CHAPTER 2

The Blood

Blood is a liquid connective tissue. It is constantly circulated from the heart to the arteries and returned back through the veins. It constitutes about 7% of total body weight and pH of blood is 7.35 to 7.45.

FUNCTIONS OF BLOOD

- **Transportation of oxygen:** The blood carries oxygen from the lungs to the tissues with the help of haemoglobin present in red blood cells.
- **Transportation of carbon dioxide:** The blood carries carbon dioxide from the tissues to excrete from the lungs.
- **Transportation of nutrients:** Blood carries the nutrients from the gastrointestinal tract to different parts of body for storage, assimilation and synthesis of new components.
- **Transportation of waste products:** Blood transports excretory products from all over the body to kidney for excretion.
- **Distribution of hormones:** Hormones produced by endocrine glands are transported by blood and distributed to their target organs.
- **Formation of clots:** Blood forms a clot following an injury to prevent further loss of blood through ruptured blood vessels.

- **Prevention of infection:** White blood cell plays a very important role in the prevention of infection by destroying bacteria.

COMPOSITION OF BLOOD

Blood consists of plasma and three different kinds of cells or corpuscles (Fig. 2.1).

Plasma

- It is a clear, straw-coloured liquid.
- The constituents of plasma are water (90–92%) and dissolved or suspended substances such as:
  - Plasma protein
    - Albumin (54%)
    - Globulin (36%)
    - Fibrinogen (7%)
    - Clotting factors
  - Inorganic salts
  - Nutrients principally from digested foods
  - Waste materials for excretion through kidneys and lungs
  - Hormones

Red Blood Cells

- Red blood cells are also called erythrocytes.
- They are biconcave, disc-like structures without any nucleus.

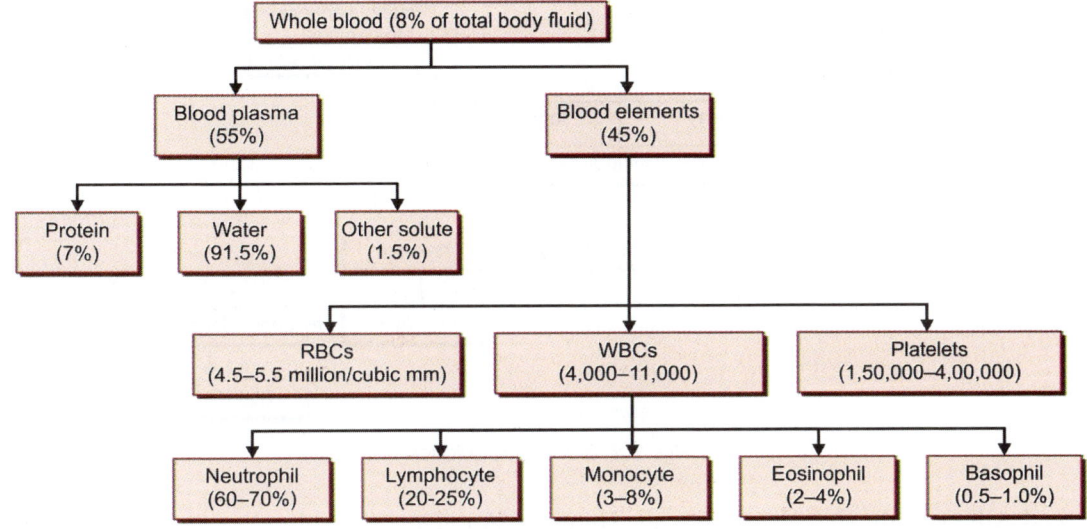

Fig. 2.1: Composition of blood

- It contains a red pigment called haemoglobin. Haemoglobin combines with oxygen at alveoli where oxygen concentration is high. At lower concentrations of oxygen at the tissue level, oxyhaemoglobin breaks and releases oxygen.
- There are five and a half million RBCs in a cubic millimetre of blood.
- Lifespan of an RBC is 120 days.
- Haematocrit is the total percentage of blood volume occupied by red blood cells.
- Normal haematocrit is 47% (40–54%) in male and 42% (38–46%) in female.

White Blood Cells

- White blood cells are also known as leucocytes.
- These cells possess a nucleus but no haemoglobin.
- They play an important role in body defence mechanism by:
  - Formation of antibodies
  - Fighting against germs
  - Ingesting and destroying bacteria (phagocytosis)

- Leucocytes are classified in two types:
  - Agranular leucocyte
    - Monocytes
    - Lymphocytes
  - Granular leucocyte
    - Neutrophils
    - Eosinophils
    - Basophils

Platelets

- Platelets are also known as thrombocytes.
- They are non-nucleated irregular shaped cell.
- Lifespan of platelet is 8–11 days.
- They prevent blood loss by the formation of a platelet plug at the site of injury.

HAEMOSTASIS

Bleeding takes place following the injury of blood vessels. Subsequently bleeding stops due to haemostasis, this consists of a series of action (Fig. 2.2).

- **Vasoconstriction:** Platelets come in contact with damaged blood vessels, become sticky

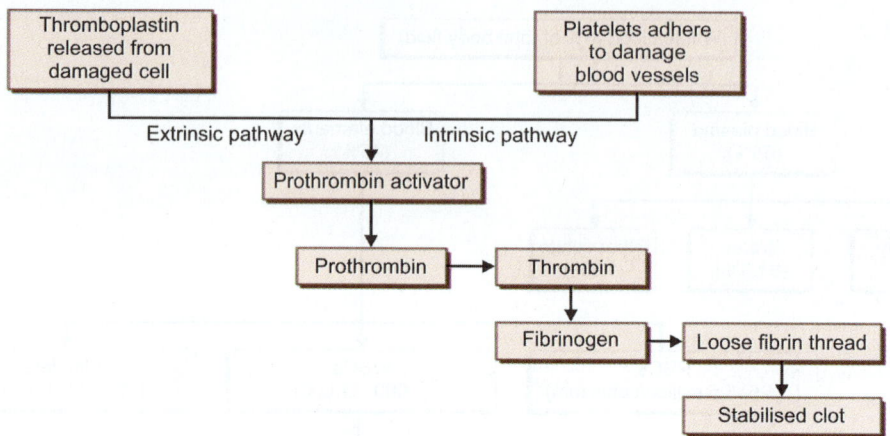

Fig. 2.2: Blood coagulation

and adhere to the damaged cell wall. They also liberate serotonin and produce vaso-constriction.

- **Platelet plug formation:** Adherent platelets liberate ADP, which attract more platelets and form a platelet plug. This plug seals the injury site.

- **Coagulation:** A number of clotting factors activate each other in a specific order as shown in Figure 2.2. Finally, fibrin is formed which stabilizes the platelet plug.

BLOOD GROUPS

Surface of the red blood cells carries different types of proteins, called antigen. These antigens are inherited and determine the blood group of an individual. There are also specific molecules in the plasma called antibodies, which are specific for a particular antigen. When a foreign antigen enters into the body, it reacts with the corresponding antibody and the antigen–antibody reaction takes place.

ABO Grouping

- Based on the type of antigen present on the surface of red blood cells, the entire population is divided into 4 types of blood group. They are group A, B, AB and O.

- A person with blood group A has antigen A on RBCs, group B has antigen B, group AB has antigens A and B and, group O has no antigen.

- If an antigen presents in RBCs, the corresponding antibody cannot be present in plasma, otherwise antigen–antibody reaction takes place and produces clumping of RBCs. Therefore, blood group 'A' person has 'b' antibody, blood group 'B' person has 'a' antibody. A person with AB group does not have antibody and 'O' group has both antibodies 'a' and 'b'.

Rh Grouping

Depending upon the presence or absence of Rhesus antigen on the red cell membrane, blood may be Rh +ve group or Rh –ve group.

BLOOD TRANSFUSION

This is a process of receiving blood or blood products by intravenous route.

Indications

- To replace blood lost during surgery or a serious injury.

- To restore the oxygen-carrying capacity of the blood.

- To prevent or treat bleeding associated with thrombocytopenia (platelet deficiency) or coagulopathy.
- To transfuse blood, if bone marrow is not producing adequate blood components due to some illness.

Procedure of Blood Transfusion

- Explain the procedure and take informed consent.
- Record baseline vital parameters.
- Check the blood bag for an identification number, ABO group and Rh compatibility report.
- Check the name of the patient, registration number and date of expiry.
- Blood or blood products must be checked and identified by two experts.
- Establish intravenous cannulation and infuse normal saline.
- Connect with blood bag and adjust the flow to deliver blood at a calculated rate.
- Watch for the signs of transfusion reactions such as fever, chills, wheezing. If transfusion reactions appear, record vital signs and stop further transfusion.
- If there is no such reaction within 15 minutes, transfusion may be continued at a predetermined rate.
- Record vital signs at the end of the procedure.

BLOOD DISORDERS

1. **Anaemia:** Anaemia is the inability of the blood to carry enough oxygen to fulfil the requirement of entire body. This is due to low level of haemoglobin or faulty haemoglobin.
2. **Polycythaemia:** A clinical condition associated with large number of red blood cells in blood. This increases blood viscosity, slows blood flow and increases the risk of intravenous clotting.
3. **Leucopaenia:** Leucopenia means white blood cells less than $4,000/mm^3$. It may occur following severe microbial infections or due to irradiation or ingestion of cytotoxic drugs.
4. **Leucocytosis:** Leucocyte count increases in response to any acute or chronic infections, which returns to normal following control of infection.
   When leucocyte count is persistently raised without any body-protective reaction, it is called leucocytosis.
5. **Leukaemia:** It is a malignant proliferation of white blood cell precursors by the bone marrow. It may be acute myeloblastic leukaemia, acute lymphoblastic leukaemia, chronic myeloid leukaemia or chronic lymphatic leukaemia.
6. **Thrombocytopaenia:** Platelet count less than $1,50,000/mm^3$ is called thrombocytopaenia. Spontaneous capillary bleeding associated with thrombocytopaenia only occurs when platelet count drops down to $30,000/mm^3$ or less.

CHAPTER 3

The Cardiovascular System

The cardiovascular system consists of two main parts:

- **The heart:** To pump and circulate blood in the whole body.
- **The blood vessels:** To carry blood for exchange of nutrients, gases and waste products.

THE HEART

- The heart is a cone-shaped hollow muscular pumping organ.
- It is located in the mediastinum of the thoracic cavity.
- The apex is about 9 cm from the midline in the left fifth intercostal space.
- The weight of adult heart is about 300 grams in male and 250 grams in female.

Position and Relations with Surrounding Structures

- **Superiorly:** Great blood vessels, aorta, superior vena cava, pulmonary artery and pulmonary veins
- **Inferiorly:** Central tendon of the diaphragm
- **Anteriorly:** Sternum, ribs and intercostal muscles

- **Posteriorly:** Oesophagus, trachea, left and right bronchi, descending aorta, inferior vena cava and thoracic vertebrae
- **Laterally:** Lungs

Structure of Heart

A. The heart wall is composed of three layers of tissues—pericardium, myocardium and endocardium.

- *Pericardium* is the outer covering membrane of the heart and is made up of two sacs. Outer sac consists of fibrous tissues and inner sac consists of two layers of serous membrane.
- *Myocardium* is the middle layer of the heart and is consisting of specialized cardiac muscles.
- *Endocardium* is the thin smooth membranous innermost layer. It ensures smooth flow of blood through the heart.

B. The heart consists of four chambers. The upper two chambers constitute the right and left atria. The lower two chambers form left and right ventricles. One-way atrioventricular valves are present between atria and ventricles, which prevent the backward flow of blood (Fig. 3.1).

Right pulmonary artery
Left pulmonary artery
Aorta
Superior vena cava
Left pulmonary veins
LA
RA
Inferior vena cava
LV
RV

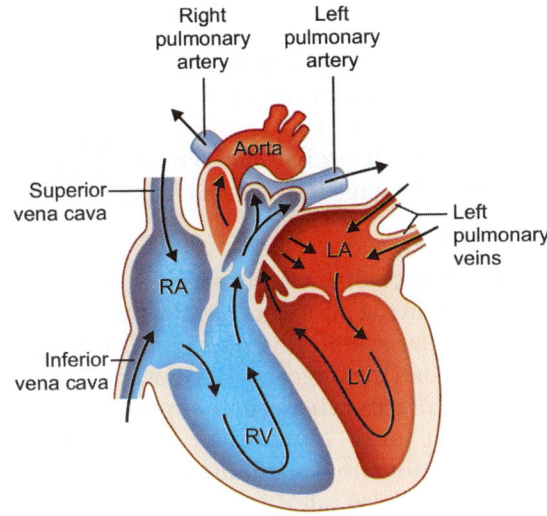

Fig. 3.1: Structure of heart

- Tricuspid valve presents between the right atrium and right ventricle.
- Bicuspid valve presents between the left atrium and left ventricle.
- Aortic valves are located at the origin of the aorta.
- Pulmonary valves present at the origin of pulmonary artery (Fig. 3.2).

Blood is pumped out from the left ventricle to the aorta, which supplies oxygenated blood to all over body through different arteries. Deoxygenated blood is collected by veins and ultimately returned to the right atrium via superior and inferior vena cava (Fig. 3.2).

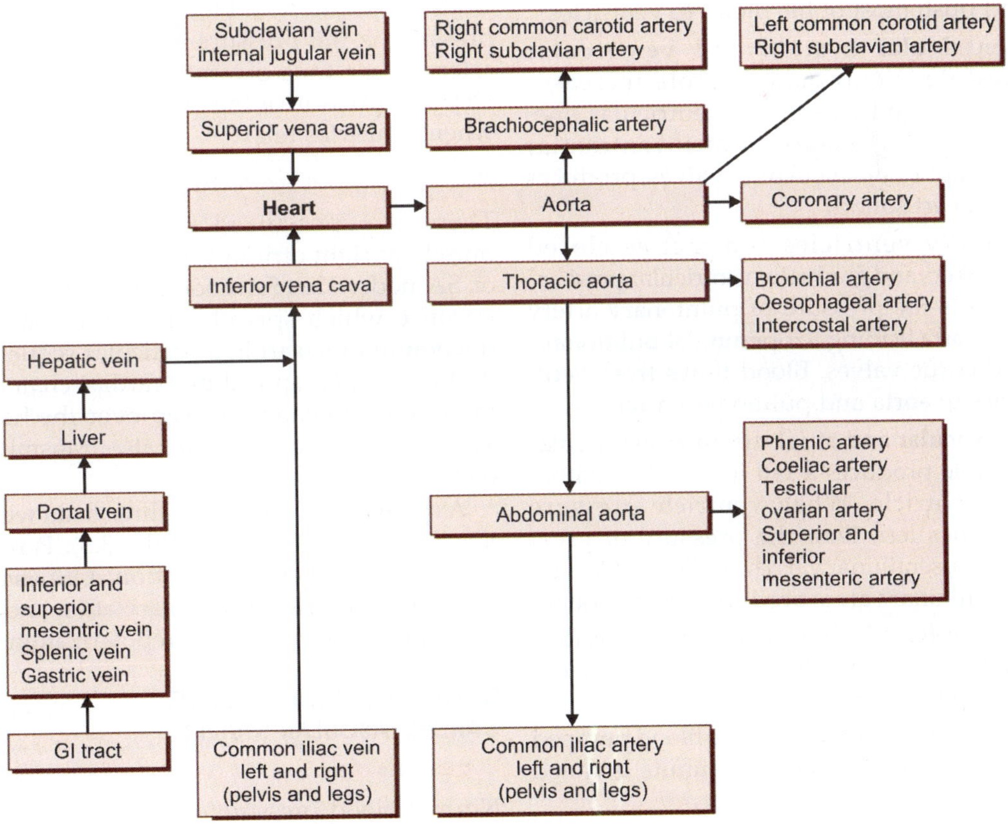

Subclavian vein internal jugular vein
Right common carotid artery Right subclavian artery
Left common corotid artery Right subclavian artery
Superior vena cava
Brachiocephalic artery
Heart
Aorta
Coronary artery
Inferior vena cava
Thoracic aorta
Bronchial artery Oesophageal artery Intercostal artery
Hepatic vein
Liver
Portal vein
Phrenic artery Coeliac artery Testicular ovarian artery Superior and inferior mesenteric artery
Abdominal aorta
Inferior and superior mesentric vein Splenic vein Gastric vein
GI tract
Common iliac vein left and right (pelvis and legs)
Common iliac artery left and right (pelvis and legs)

Fig. 3.2: Circulation of blood: Aorta, vena cava and their main branches

Function of the Heart

Rhythmic contraction and relaxation of the cardiac chamber in a particular sequence cause forward propulsion of blood. On an average, heart contracts and relaxes 70 to 80 times/minute and pumps about 5 liters of blood per minute.

Contraction of the cardiac chamber is called systole and relaxation is called diastole.

1. **Atrial filling and joint diastole:** Due to atrial relaxation, blood flows from superior and inferior vena cava to the right atrium and from pulmonary vein to left atrium.

   Pressure within the atrium increases due to filling of blood and opens one-way valve (tricuspid and bicuspid). Blood flows from atrium to ventricles.

2. **Atrial systole and ventricular diastole:** At the end of the joint diastole, atria contract and push most of the blood to ventricles.

3. **Ventricular systole and ventricular diastole:** Ventricular systole increases pressure and closes atrioventricular one-way valve. Closure of atrioventricular (tricuspid and bicuspid) valves produces first heart sound.

   Initially ventricles contract as closed chambers and gradually ventricular pressure exceeds the pressure of pulmonary artery and aorta leading to opening of pulmonary and aortic valves. Blood flows from ventricles to aorta and pulmonary artery.

4. **Ventricular and atrial diastole:** Ventricular diastole produces a fall in pressure within the ventricle. When ventricle pressure becomes less than the pressure of great vessels, semilunar valves are closed. Closure of semilunar valves produces second sound.

   Stroke volume: Volume of the blood pumped out by each ventricle in one cardiac cycle is called stroke volume.

   Cardiac output: Volume of the blood pumped out by each ventricle per minute is called cardiac output.

   Cardiac output = Stroke volume × number of heart beats per minute

Heart Beat

Closure of atrioventricular valves and semilunar valves produces first and second sounds—lub dub. This sound is reflected as heart beat. Each cardiac cycle constitutes one heart beat. Average heart beat is 72 per minute.

Pulse Rate

It is a wave of distension followed by constriction felt in the peripheral arteries as a result of ventricular systole and diastole. This is felt as pulse when the finger is placed on the artery at certain places where, it is superficial like near wrist joint. Number of beats felt at peripheral pulse in one minute is counted and recorded as pulse rate.

Blood Pressure

The pressure exerted by the blood against the walls of the arteries is blood pressure. Systolic pressure is the pressure experienced in the artery at the time of ventricular contraction. Diastolic pressure is the pressure in the artery when ventricles relax.

Electrocardiogram (ECG)

There is a specialized area in the cardiac muscle of right atrium called sinoatrial node or SA node. This SA node generates cardiac impulse which spreads as a wave of contraction in the heart in a particular sequence. As this impulse spread in a cardiac chamber, the electrical changes sweep over the heart. These electrical changes are also transmitted on the surface of the body.

A normal ECG consists of three main waves 'P', 'QRS' and, 'T' waves (Fig. 3.3). P wave indicates atrial depolarization, QRS wave represents ventricular depolarization and 'T' wave indicates ventricular repolarization.

DISORDERS RELATED TO THE CARDIOVASCULAR SYSTEM

Hypertension

Normal blood pressure of an adult is about 120/80 mm Hg. When blood pressure is more than 140/90 mm Hg, it is called hypertension.

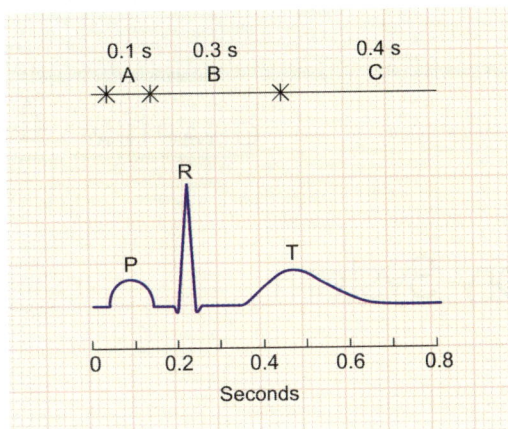

Fig. 3.3: Normal ECG

Coronary Artery Disease

There is insufficient blood supply to the heart muscles due to atherosclerosis of the coronary artery.

Insufficiency of blood supply leads to chest pain or angina. Complete block of coronary artery produces myocardial infarction or heart attack.

Heart Failure

A clinical condition when heart is not able to pump blood effectively enough to meet the need of the body is also called congestive heart failure because it causes congestion in the lungs.

CHAPTER 4

The Respiratory System

The respiratory system is a channel for gaseous exchange between atmosphere, blood and cells.

ORGANS OF THE RESPIRATORY SYSTEM

The respiratory system consists of:

- Upper respiratory system
  - Nose
  - Pharynx
- Lower respiratory system
  - Larynx
  - Trachea
  - Bronchi
  - Alveoli

Nose and Nasal Cavity

The nasal cavity is a large irregular space divided into two equal parts by a septum. It is lined with very vascular ciliated columnar epithelium which secretes mucous for moistening the cavity. It is connected to the exterior by two nostrils.

Functions

- Filtration of inhaled air
- Moisturization and warming of inhaled air
- Detection of smell (olfactory stimuli)

Pharynx

The pharynx is a cavity at the back of the mouth and nasal cavity. It is a common passage for food and air.

Parts of Pharynx

- Nasopharynx
- Oropharynx
- Laryngopharynx

Functions

- It acts as a passage for air and food.
- The air is warmed and humidified as it passes through the pharynx.
- Pharynx is also involved in speech.
- The lymphatic tissue of pharyngeal tonsils produces antibodies in response to swallowed or inhaled antigens (microorganisms).

Larynx

Larynx is also known as voice box. It connects laryngopharynx to trachea. The larynx is composed of epiglottis, thyroid cartilage, cricoid cartilage and a pair of arytenoid cartilages. They are attached to each other by ligaments and membranes.

There are two pale folds arise from thyroid cartilage called vocal cords. Different sounds can be produced by varying degree of tension of vocal cords.

Functions

- Sound and speech production.
- Protection of respiratory passage.
- Humidification, filtering and warming of the air.

Trachea, Bronchus and Bronchioles

- Trachea extends downwards from larynx to 5th thoracic vertebra where it divides into two branches right bronchus and left bronchus.
- Right and left bronchi further divide into secondary and tertiary bronchi.
- The terminal bronchi divide and subdivide into bronchioles, terminal bronchioles, respiratory bronchioles, alveolar ducts and alveoli.

Functions

- Cough reflex
- Warming and humidification of air
- Mucociliary escalator for upwards movements of particles which are subsequently either swallowed or coughed out.

LUNGS

- There are two lungs located in the right side and left side of the thoracic cavity. Each lung is enclosed in a double-walled sac called pleura.
- Right lobe is divided into three lobes—superior lobe, middle lobe and inferior lobe. Left lung is divided into superior lobe and inferior lobe.
- Both lungs contain about 300 million alveoli. They are thin-walled air sac covered by blood capillaries. Respiratory gases are exchanged between the blood and alveolar air by diffusion through the alveolar wall.
- Total surface area of alveoli available for gas exchange is approximately 400–800 square feet.

Respiration

- Respiration means exchange of gases between the body cells and atmosphere.
- It includes following processes:
  - Breathing or movement of air in and out of the lungs
  - Exchange of gases
    - In the lungs—external respiration
    - In the tissues—internal respiration

Breathing

- Breathing process consists of inspiration, expiration and expiratory pause.
- During inspiration, the air is inhaled from the atmosphere.
- During expiration, expired gases are exhaled from the lungs.
- Breathing is a process of in and out of the air from the lungs.
- Normal adult breath 12–14 breaths per minute.

Lung Volumes and Capacities (Fig. 4.1)

1. **Tidal volume (TV):** It is the volume of air breathed in and out during each cycle of breathing. (Tidal volume – 500 ml)
2. **Inspiratory reserve volume (IRV):** It is the extra volume of air over and above the tidal volume that can be breath in during deep inspiration. (IRV = 2500 to 3000 ml)
3. **Expiratory reserve volume (ERV):** Maximum volume of air which can be expelled from the lungs after a normal expiration. (ERV = 1000 to 1100 ml)
4. **Residual volume (RV):** Volume of air remaining in the lungs even after the maximum expiration is called residual volume. Residual volume of air is always present in the lungs. (RV = 1100 to 1200 ml)
5. **Inspiratory capacity (IC):** Maximum volume of air which can be breath in is called inspiratory capacity. (IC = TV + IRV = 3000 to 3500 ml)

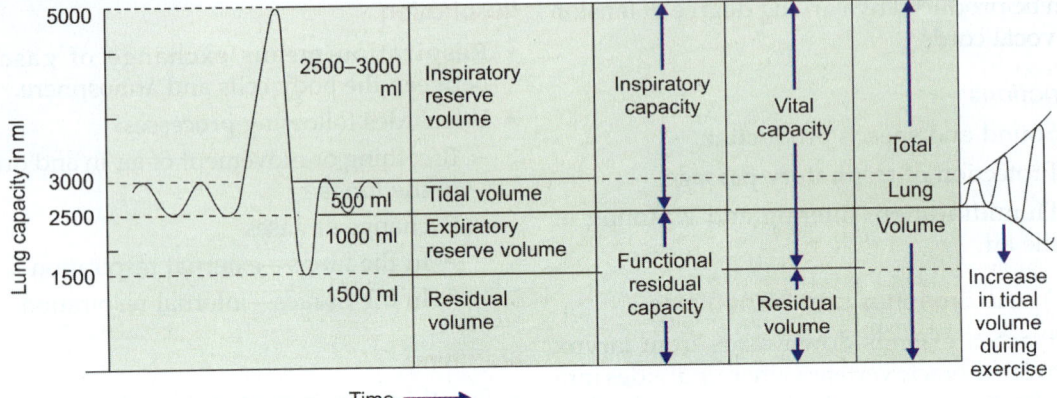

Fig. 4.1: Lung volumes and capacities

6. **Expiratory capacity (EC):** Maximum volume of air which can be expired after a normal inspiration. (EC = TV + ERV = 1500 to 2000 ml)

7. **Functional residual capacity (FRC):** Volume of air that remains in the lungs after a normal expiration is called functional residual capacity. (FRC = ERV + RV = 1100+1100 = 2200)

8. **Vital capacity (VC):** Volume of air expired after a maximum inspiration followed by a maximum expiration. (VC = IRV+ TV + ERV = 4000 to 4500 ml)

9. **Total lung capacity (TLC):** Volume of air presents in the lungs after the maximum inspiration. (TLC = VC+RV = 5500 to 6000 ml)

10. **Dead space:** Volume of air present in the respiratory tubes where gaseous exchange does not take place. It is approximately one-third of the tidal volume, i.e. 150 ml for a normal adult male.

EXCHANGE OF GASES

Exchange of oxygen and carbon dioxide at the respiratory alveoli and in the tissues is a continuous process. Diffusion of oxygen and carbon dioxide across the membrane depends on the pressure differences between the atmospheric air and blood or blood and the tissues (Table 4.1).

External Respiration

Exchange of gases across the alveolar membrane between the alveoli and the blood in alveolar capillaries is called external respiration.

Venous blood from all over the body reaches the lungs via the pulmonary artery. This deoxygenated blood has a low level of oxygen and a high level of carbon dioxide. Therefore, depending upon the concentration gradient, oxygen diffuses from the alveoli into the blood till the equilibrium occurs. Similarly, carbon dioxide diffuses across the alveolar

Table 4.1	Partial pressure of gases at different level (mm Hg)				
Respiratory gas	Atmospheric air	Alveoli	Pulmonary artery (deoxygenated blood)	Pulmonary vein (oxygenated blood)	Tissues
PO_2	159	104	40	95	40
PCO_2	0.3	40	45	40	45

membrane from deoxygenated blood to alveoli. Partial pressure of oxygen and carbon dioxide in the blood leaving the alveolar capillary is same as the alveolar gas.

Internal Respiration

Exchange of gases between the capillary blood and tissues is called internal respiration. Blood at the arterial end of capillaries has a higher PO_2 and lower PCO_2 than the tissue. Therefore, gas exchange takes place due to these concentration gradients.

Oxygen diffuses from blood to the tissue and carbon dioxide diffuses from tissue to blood across the capillary membrane.

TRANSPORT OF GASES IN BLOOD

Blood transports oxygen from lungs to different tissues and carbon dioxide from the tissues to the lungs.

Oxygen

Transport of oxygen in the blood takes place by two ways.

1. It combines with haemoglobin to form oxyhaemoglobin (98.5%)

$$Hb + 4O_2 \underset{\text{Tissues}}{\overset{\text{Lugs}}{\rightleftarrows}} Hb\,(4O_2)$$

2. Approximately 1.5% of oxygen is carried as a solution by dissolving in plasma.

Oxyhaemoglobin dissociates and releases oxygen in presence of low O_2 level, low pH, raised temperature and high CO_2 level.

Carbon Dioxide

Carbon dioxide is produced in the tissues as a waste product and is transported to the lungs by three mechanisms.

1. As carbonic acid in the plasma (7%). Carbon dioxide combines with water to form carbonic acid and carried by plasma in solution form.

$$CO_2 + H_2O \rightarrow H_2CO_3$$

2. As carbaminohaemoglobin in the RBCs (23%). Carbon dioxide enters into the RBCs and forms a reversible compound with amino group of globin of reduced haemoglobin.

$$HNbNH_2 + CO_2 \rightarrow HbNHCOOH + H^+$$

3. As bicarbonate ions (HCO_3^-) in the plasma (70%). A major part of carbon dioxide enters in the red blood cells and rapidly converted to the carbonic acid in presence of enzyme carbonic anhydrase. Carbonic acid dissociates into bicarbonates (HCO_3^-) and hydrogen (H^+) ions. Some of the bicarbonate ions diffuse out into plasma, where they combine with sodium ions to form sodium bicarbonate.

DISORDERS OF THE RESPIRATORY SYSTEM

Upper Respiratory Tract Infections

Upper respiratory tract infections are usually viral in origin. Viruses lower the resistance of the respiratory tract and allow the bacteria to invade the tissue. Viral infection causes tissue congestion and profuse watery secretions. Secretion becomes purulent, if the secondary bacterial infection takes place.

- Common cold is caused by rhinoviruses and influenza by a different group of viruses. They affect nose and pharynx and cause rhinorrhoea, sneezing, sore throat and, fever. Spontaneous recovery takes place in one week provided secondary bacterial infections do not occur.
- Infections may spread from the upper respiratory tract to larynx and trachea and produce laryngitis and tracheitis.

Bronchitis

- Acute bronchitis is usually due to secondary bacterial infections. Chronic bronchitis is due to pollutants like smoke or carbon dioxide. It causes frequent coughing with heavy mucous discharge.
- Best preventive measure is to avoid exposure to pollutant.

- Treatment consists of:
  - Antibiotics to control infection
  - Bronchodilator to widen the constricted bronchial passage.

Bronchial Asthma

- It is the hypersensitivity of the bronchioles to certain allergic substances.
- It produces spasm of smooth muscles of bronchioles leading to cough, difficulty in breathing mainly during expiration and excessive secretions.
- Treatment consists of antibiotics and bronchodilator inhalation.

Emphysema

- Chronic exposure of lung tissues to smoke and air pollutants leads to the destruction of lung tissue along with abnormal distension of alveolar sacs.
- It is a chronic obstructive lung disease, presented with chronic cough and breathlessness.
- Bronchodilators, antibiotics, oxygen therapy and chest physiotherapy may slow the progress of the disease.

Pneumonia

- Acute infection of alveoli by bacteria, most common *Streptococcus pneumoniae*.
- It can be viral, fungal or protozoal in origin.
- Treatment includes antibiotics to control infection and bronchodilator drugs to decrease respiratory distress.

Bronchial Carcinoma

- It is a very common malignancy and has a close association with smoking.
- As the tumour grows within the bronchus, it may produce signs of obstruction.
- Treatment includes chemotherapy, radiotherapy, immunotherapy and surgery.

CHAPTER 5

The Digestive System

The digestive system consists of the alimentary canal and its accessory organs which are responsible for ingestion, digestion, assimilation and removal of the undigested waste materials.

ALIMENTARY CANAL

Alimentary canal starts from the mouth and ends at the anus. It is a long coiled muscular tube of about nine metres in length.

It includes following organs (Fig. 5.1)**:**
- Mouth
- Pharynx
- Oesophagus
- Stomach
- Small intestine
- Large intestine
- Rectum and anal canal

Associated Digestive Organs

Apart from a large number of gastric and intestinal glands, there are three main digestive glands, which are closely associated with the digestive process. They are:
- Salivary glands
- Liver and biliary tract
- Pancreas

Basic Structure of the Alimentary Tract

The walls of the alimentary tract are formed by four-level of tissue:
- Adventitia or serosa
- Muscle
- Submucosa
- Mucosa

Adventitia or Serosa

This is the outmost layer of the alimentary tract. In the thorax, it consists of loose fibrous tissue. In the abdomen, it is a serous membrane called peritoneum. Peritoneum is the largest serous membrane of the body. It consists of two layers.

1. Outer parietal peritoneum lines the abdominal wall.
2. Inner visceral peritoneal covers the organs within abdominal and pelvic cavities.

It is a closed sac which acts as a physical barrier for the spread of infection from one organ to other organ. It isolates the infective focus and protects other organs.

Muscle Layer

- It consists of two layers of smooth muscle—the inner circular layer and outer longitudinal layer. An oblique muscle layer may be present in some regions.

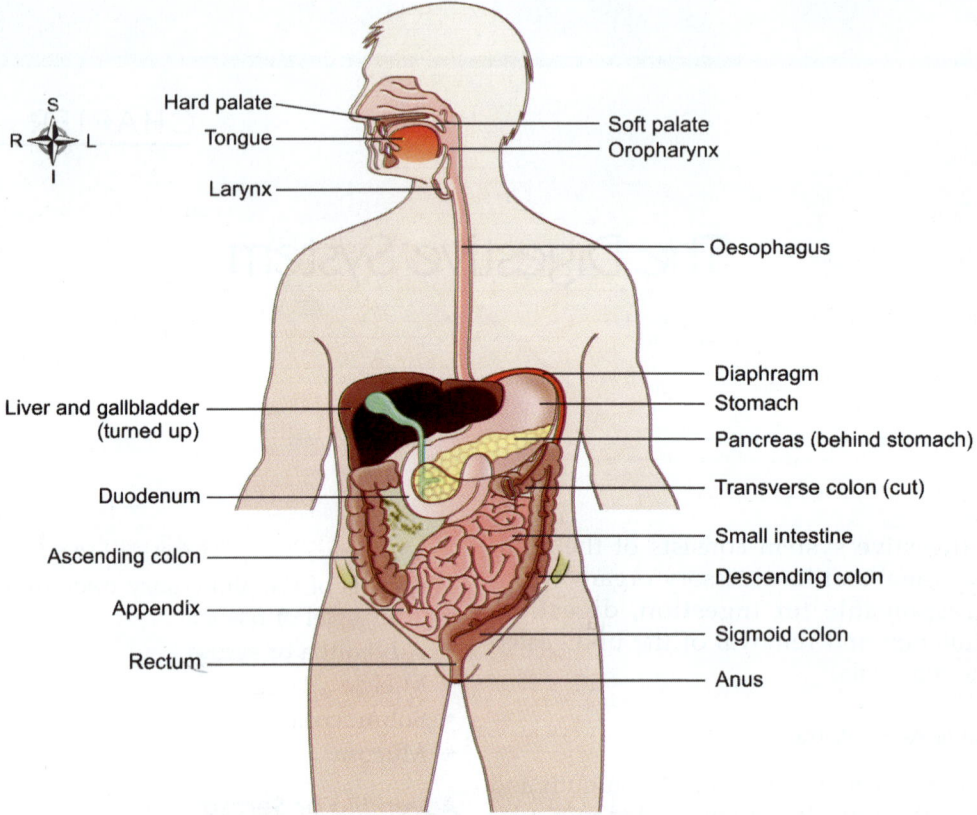

Fig. 5.1: Digestive system

- Contractions and relaxations of these muscles lead to the forward movement of content within the alimentary canal.
- Circular muscle becomes thick at various points and forms sphincters. They regulate the movements of content within the alimentary canal.

Submucosa

This consists of loose areolar connective tissue, blood vessels, nerves and lymph vessels are present within this layer.

Mucosa

- Mucosa consists of three layers:
  a. Mucous membrane consists of columnar epithelium.
  b. Lamina propria consists of loose connective tissue

c. Muscularis mucosa consists of a thin layer of smooth muscle which is responsible for involutions of the mucosal layer.

- Mucosa is the innermost lining of the alimentary tract.
- Mucosa provides protection, secretes mucous as well as digestive juices by specialized cells and absorbs digested food materials.
- Secretions of digestive juices in the lumen of the alimentary tract include:
  - Saliva from salivary glands
  - Gastric juice from gastric glands
  - Intestinal juice from intestinal glands
  - Pancreatic juice from pancreas
  - Bile from liver.

Nerve Supply

Parasympathetic Nerve

One pair of vagus cranial nerves supplies most of the alimentary tract. Distal parts of the tract are supplied by sacral nerves.

Sympathetic Nerve

Nerves from the spinal cord in thoracic and lumbar regions form plexus and supply organs of the alimentary tract.

Parts of Alimentary Canal

Oral or Buccal Cavity

Oral cavity (Fig. 5.2) is bounded by muscles and bones.
- Anteriorly—by the lips
- Posteriorly—continues with the oropharynx
- Laterally—by cheeks
- Superiorly—by bony hard palate (anterior part) and soft muscular palate (posterior part).
- Uvula is a curved fold, hanging down from the middle of the free border of the soft palate.

- Inferiorly—by tongue and soft tissue of the floor of the mouth

Pharynx

Posteriorly oral and nasal cavities continue as pharynx. This again divided into two parts: Anteriorly wind pipe called larynx and trachea and posteriorly food pipe as oesophagus.

Oesophagus

It is a straight muscular tube, transports food from mouth to stomach. It passes through the neck, thorax and diaphragm and opens in the stomach.

Stomach

It is a large musculoelastic bag situated below the diaphragm. It has three parts—fundus, cardia and pylorus. Stomach squeezes and churns the food and mixed with gastric juice secreted by gastric glands. Pyloric sphincter is situated at the outlet of stomach. It acts as a valve and does not open until food is fully mixed and churned.

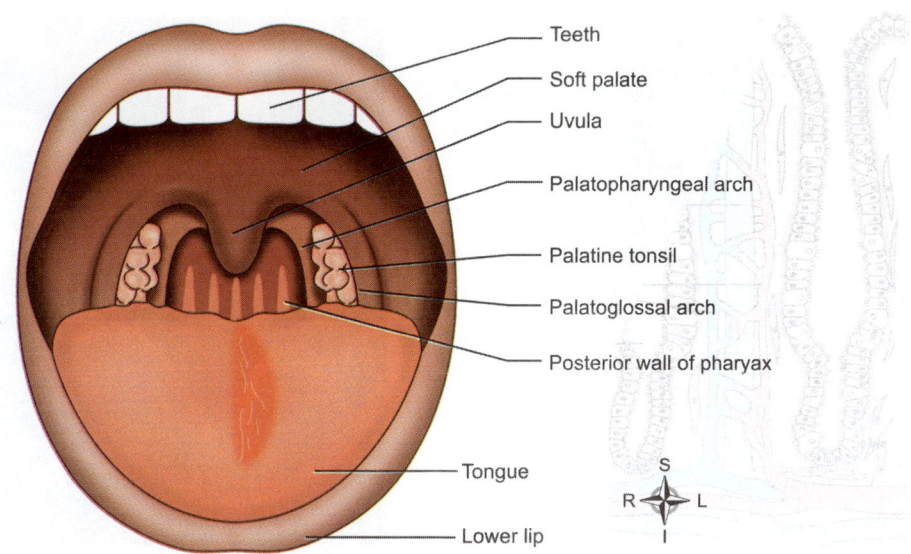

Teeth
Soft palate
Uvula
Palatopharyngeal arch
Palatine tonsil
Palatoglossal arch
Posterior wall of pharyax
Tongue
Lower lip

Fig. 5.2: Oral cavity

Small Intestine

It consists of three parts—duodenum, jejunum and ileum.

- *Duodenum* is the upper part of the small intestine. It is 'C' shaped and receive pancreatic juice from pancreas and bile juice from the liver through gall bladder and common bile ducts.
- Duodenum opens into a coiled tube called *jejunum* which ultimately leads to ileum.
- *Ileum* is a highly coiled tubular structure. Inner wall has a number of finger-like projections called villi. It increases the surface area for absorption. In between the villi, there are glandular pits which secrete the digestive enzyme (Fig. 5.3A and B).

Large Intestine

Large intestine consists of three parts—caecum, colon and rectum.

- *Caecum* is a sac-like structure, proximally connected to the ileum and distally continued as colon. It has a finger-like projection called appendix.
- *Colon* consists of ascending colon, transverse colon, descending colon and pelvic colon. It is located as inverted 'U' shaped in the abdominal cavity. Food can remain in colon for a long time.
- Absorption of water takes place and finally waste material is formed to eliminate from the body.
- *Rectum* is the last part of large intestine. External opening of rectum is called anus. Anal sphincter consisting of circular muscle, is present at the anal opening and responsible for the closure of anus.

ASSOCIATED DIGESTIVE ORGANS

Salivary Glands

There are three pairs of salivary glands—parotid, submaxillary and sublingual. They secrete saliva into the mouth. Saliva not only lubricates food and helps in swallowing but also helps in digestion of starch by an enzyme salivary amylase.

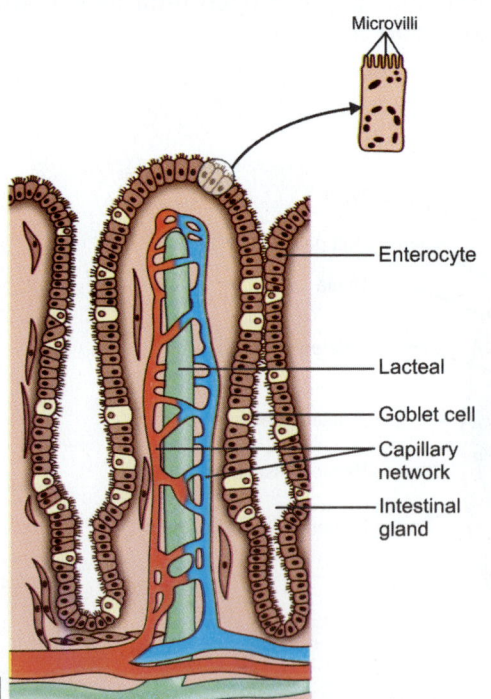

Microvilli

Enterocyte

Lacteal

Goblet cell

Capillary network

Intestinal gland

A

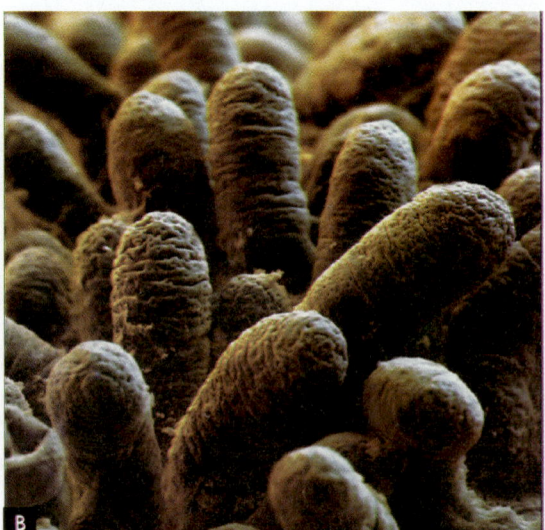

B

Fig. 5.3A and B: Villus of the small intestine

Pancreas

- It is located in the bend of the duodenal loop.
- It has dual functions—exocrine and endocrine.
- Exocrine part secretes pancreatic juice containing three enzymes; lipase, trypsin and amylase to act on fats, proteins and starch respectively.
- Pancreatic duct joins the common bile duct to form hepatopancreatic duct and finally opens into the duodenum. Opening is guarded by a sphincter called sphincter of Oddi.

Liver

Liver is the largest gland of the body, located mainly at right upper quadrant of the abdominal cavity.

Bile juice, secreted by liver, is passed through hepatic duct and stored in the gallbladder. Gallbladder and bile duct are located at the under surface of the liver. Hepatic duct and bile duct join and form common bile duct. Gallbladder concentrates bile and releases into the duodenum during the process of digestion.

Functions of Liver

- Formation of bile and bile salt
- Regulation of blood sugar
- Production of blood clotting factor, fibrinogen
- Production of heparin
- Storage of fat-soluble vitamins A and D
- Storage of iron
- Deamination of excess amino acids and conversion into urea.

DIGESTION OF FOOD

Digestion at Oral Cavity

Digestion of food starts from the oral cavity. Ingested food is chewed by teeth and broken into small particles. The food is mixed with saliva and digestive process starts by following ways.

- Salivary amylase breaks starch into maltose, a disaccharide

$$\text{Starch} \xrightarrow{\text{Salivary amylase}} \text{Maltose + Isomaltose} + \text{Limit dextrins}$$

- Mucous moistens and dissolves some food and lubricates the oesophagus.
- Bicarbonate ions neutralize acids in food.
- Thiocyanate ions act as an antimicrobial agent and prevent infection by a microorganism.
- Lysozyme kills bacteria and prevents infections.

Digestion in Stomach

Gastric muscle generates a churning action and breaks down the bolus of ingested food and mixes it with gastric juice. Gastric juice consists of hydrochloric acid, mucous and pepsinogen.

Hydrochloric Acid

- Brings the pH of the stomach between 1.5 and 2.5.
- Kills germs and bacteria.
- Inactivates salivary amylase and prevents further breakdown of carbohydrate by amylase.
- Convert inactive pepsinogen into pepsin.

Mucus

It acts as a lubricant and protects the lining of stomach.

Pepsinogen

It gets converted into protein digestive enzyme, pepsin in the presence of hydrochloric acid.

$$\text{Pepsinogen} \xrightarrow{\text{HCl}} \text{Pepsin}$$

$$\text{Pepsinogen} \xrightarrow{\text{Pepsin}} \text{Pepsin}$$

$$\text{Proteins} \xrightarrow{\text{Pepsin}} \text{Short peptides}$$

Stomach also produces intrinsic factor which helps in absorption of vitamin B_{12}. Stomach converts food into a semiliquid mass, called chyme. This semiliquid mass enters into the duodenum through the pyloric sphincter.

Digestion in Small Intestine

Duodenum receives pancreatic juice from pancreas, bile juice from liver via gallbladder and intestinal juice from the lining of the intestine.

Pancreatic Juice

- Pancreatic juice contains water, enzymes and bicarbonates. Bicarbonates neutralize the hydrochloric acid and create optimum condition for digestive enzymes.
- Pancreatic juice contains inactive form of proteolytic enzymes—trypsinogen, chymo-trypsinogen and procarboxypeptidase. It also contains pancreatic lipase and amylase.

Trypsinogen

$$\text{Trypsinogen} \xrightarrow[\text{(by intestine)}]{\text{Enterokinase}} \text{Trypsin} + \text{inactive peptide}$$

$$\text{Trypsinogen} \xrightarrow{\text{Trypsin}} \text{Trypsin}$$

$$\text{Proteins} \xrightarrow{\text{Trypsin}} \text{Polypeptides}$$

Chymotrypsinogen

$$\text{Chymotrypsinogen} \xrightarrow{\text{Trypsin}} \text{Chymotrypsin}$$

$$\text{Proteins} \xrightarrow{\text{Chymotrypsin}} \text{Polypeptides}$$

Procaboxypeptidase

$$\text{Procarboxypeptidase} \xrightarrow{\text{Trypsin}} \text{Carboxypeptidase}$$

$$\text{Polypeptides} \xrightarrow{\text{Carboxypeptidase}} \text{Peptides} + \text{amino acids}$$

Pancreatic amylase

$$\text{Starch} \xrightarrow{\text{Pancreatic amylase}} \text{Disaccharides}$$

Pancreatic lipase

$$\text{Fats} \xrightarrow{\text{Pancreatic lipase}} \text{Fatty acids} + \text{glycerol}$$

Bile Juice

Bile juice is consisting of water, bile pigments, bile salts, cholesterol and phospholipids. Bile salts play an important role in the digestion of fat. Bile salts break large fat or oil droplets into microscopic droplets and increase the surface area for the action of lipase. This process of breaking large fat droplets is called fat emulsifications.

Intestinal Juice

Intestinal juice contains digestive enzymes but they are not released into the lumen of intestine. They either act within the cell or closed to the border of the cells.

$$\text{Dipeptides} \xrightarrow{\text{Dipeptidase}} \text{Amino acids}$$

$$\text{Maltose} \xrightarrow{\text{Dipeptidase}} \text{Glucose} + \text{glucose}$$

$$\text{Lactose} \xrightarrow{\text{Lactase}} \text{Glucose} + \text{galactose}$$

$$\text{Sucrose} \xrightarrow{\text{Sucrose}} \text{Glucose} + \text{fructose}$$

$$\text{Di and mono- glycerides} \xrightarrow{\text{Lipase}} \text{Fatty acids} + \text{glycerol}$$

Thus digestion starts in the mouth and completes in the small intestine. The digested food consists of glucose, fructose, galactose, amino acids, fatty acids and glycerol. Most of the absorption of digested food materials takes place in the ileum. Large intestine is concerned with absorption of water and formation of faeces by undigested materials.

COMMON SURGICAL DISORDERS OF THE DIGESTIVE SYSTEM

Infectious and inflammatory conditions may occur in any parts of gastrointestinal tract from mouth to anal canal. Depending upon the type of infections, they usually respond to anti-bacterial or antifungal agents. Similarly malignancy can occur in any part of gastrointestinal tract.

Some of the common surgical conditions of the digestive system are as follows.

Cleft Lip and Cleft Palate

Normally roof of the mouth is formed by the fusion of two structures grown from two sides. If fusion is incomplete, a cleft at the roof of mouth persists. It may be as minor as a small notch in the upper lip or may be complete gap involving the soft and hard palate. Surgical correction is the treatment of this congenital disorders.

Peptic Ulcer

Peptic ulcer commonly occurs at the stomach and first few centimetres of the duodenum. Complications of peptic ulcer are haemorrhage, perforation, malignancy and gastric outlet obstruction. They usually require surgical interventions.

Appendicitis

Inflammation of the appendix is called appendicitis. This may lead to ischaemia, gangrene, rupture, peritonitis or abscess formation. Surgical removal of the appendix is indicated in such a scenario.

Hernia

It is protrusion of an organ or part of an organ through a weak point or aperture in the surrounding structure. Depending upon the site of protrusion of intra-abdominal organs, it may be:

- Inguinal hernia (herniation through inguinal canal)
- Femoral hernia (herniation through femoral canal)
- Umbilical hernia (herniation at umbilicus)
- Hiatus hernia (protrusion of the part of fundus of the stomach through oesophageal opening in the diaphragm)
- Incisional hernia (protrusion of abdominal organs through the weak point of the scar of previous surgery at the site of incision).

Outcome of the hernia includes: (a) Spontaneous reduction following reduction of intra-abdominal pressure, (b) manual reduction by applying gentle pressure over the swelling, or (c) strangulation when reduction is not possible. Strangulation may lead to ischaemia, intestinal obstruction and gangrene.

Volvulus

A loop of bowel twists itself, occludes the lumen of the intestine and produces intestinal obstruction. It may lead to gangrene following interruption of the blood supply.

Intussusceptions

It is invagination of a part of intestine within the lumen of adjacent intestine. End result is intestinal obstruction, ischaemia and if remain untreated, gangrene.

Intestinal Obstruction

It is the occlusion of intestinal lumen leading to prevention of forward movement of digestive materials. It is usually mechanical in origin following peritoneal adhesions, stenosis or tumour of the intestinal wall. It may be neurological in origin causes cessation of peristaltic activity (paralytic ileus).

Symptoms of intestinal obstruction include abdominal pain, vomiting and absolute constipation. It leads to dehydration, shock and electrolyte imbalance. Release of obstruction by removal of cause is the treatment of such condition.

Gallstone (Cholelithiasis)

Cholelithiasis is the formation of one or multiple stones by deposition of bile or cholesterol within the gallbladder. It may not produce any symptom unless some complications occur like cholecystitis or occlusion of the bile duct by a stone.

Surgical removal of gallbladder or cholecystectomy is indicated in such situation.

CHAPTER 6

The Musculoskeletal System

The musculoskeletal system consists of skeleton of bones, joints, and skeletal muscles.

SKELETAL SYSTEM

The skeletal system is a basic framework of the body and gives it a proper shape. It is mainly composed of bones and cartilages.

Functions of Skeletal System

- Skeletal system constitutes a rigid framework and maintains specific shape of the body.
- Skeletal system protects and supports vital organs like the brain, lungs and heart.
- Skeleton along with joints and skeletal muscles is an important constituent of locomotion and is responsible for the movement of the body.
- It acts as a storage system for calcium and phosphate.
- Red bone marrow of the bone is a haemopoietic tissue and produces red blood cells and white blood cells.

Parts of the Skeletal System (Fig. 6.1)

Skeletal system has two parts:

- *Axial skeleton* consists of skull, vertebral column, ribs and sternum.
- *Appendicular skeleton* consists of bones of the upper limb, lower limb, pectoral girdles and pelvic girdles.

Axial Skeleton

Skull

Skull rests on the upper end of the vertebral column. Skull consists of the cranium (8 bones) and facial bones (14 bones). Different parts of the skull have different functions.

- Cranium protects the brain
- Bony eye sockets protect eyes and muscular attachments help them to move in different directions.
- Temporal bone protects the inner ear.
- Bones of face and nose form the upper airway.
- Maxilla and mandible provide ridges for teeth.
- Movements of mandible produce chewing.

Cranium: The cranium is also called brain box. It consists of eight flat and slightly arched bone.

- Frontal bone—1
- Parietal bone—2
- Temporal bone—2
- Occipital bone—1
- Sphenoid bone—1
- Ethmoid bone—1

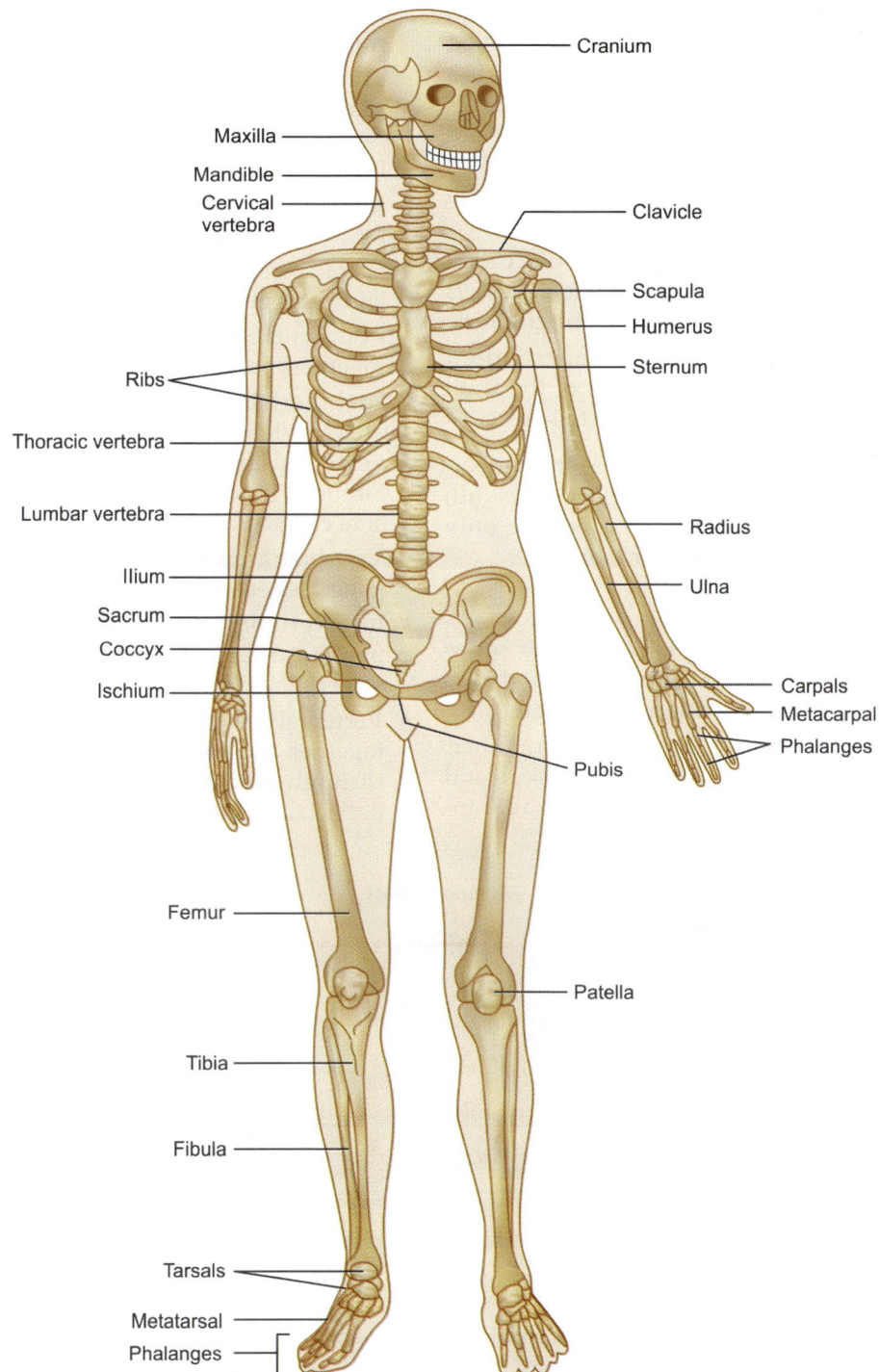

Fig. 6.1: Human skeleton

These bones are tightly interlocking with each other by their serrated margins called sutures. At the posterior lower end, there is a large opening called foramen magnum. On either side of the foramen magnum, there is a smooth rounded projection called condyle which articulates with the first cervical vertebra (atlas).

Bones have numerous perforations called foramina through which nerves, blood vessels and lymph vessels enter or leave the cranium.

Cranial bones have air spaces called sinuses. They reduce the weight of the skull and also give resonant sound to the voice.

Facial bones: Facial bones are 14 in number. They constitute the front part of the skull, nose, hard palate and lower jaw. The only movable part is lower jaw or mandible.

Vertebral Column

Vertebral column made up of a linear series of bones called vertebrae. There are 33 vertebrae basically divided into 5 types.

- Cervical vertebrae are seven in number. First vertebra, atlas, supports the skull and allows, flexion and extension at atlanto-occipital joint. Second vertebra, axis, allows rotational movements of the skull.
- Thoracic vertebrae are twelve in number. They connect with ribs and sternum to form the thoracic cage to protect the heart and lungs.
- Lumbar vertebrae are five in number and located at the lumbar region.
- Sacral vertebrae are five in number. They joined together and form sacrum.
- Four vertebrae at the tail end joined together and form coccyx or tail bone.
- Each vertebra has a body and vertebral arch. Posteriorly, there is a prominence on vertebral arch called spinous process. Similarly, there is one projection on each side called transverse process (Fig. 6.2).
- Vertebrae are arranged in a linear series and joined together by intervertebral discs.
- Intervertebral disc is made up of white fibrous cartilage. It allows limited movement of vertebrae.
- Vertebral foramen of each vertebra is joined together and forms a hollow central canal through which spinal cord passes from occipital region to coccyx.

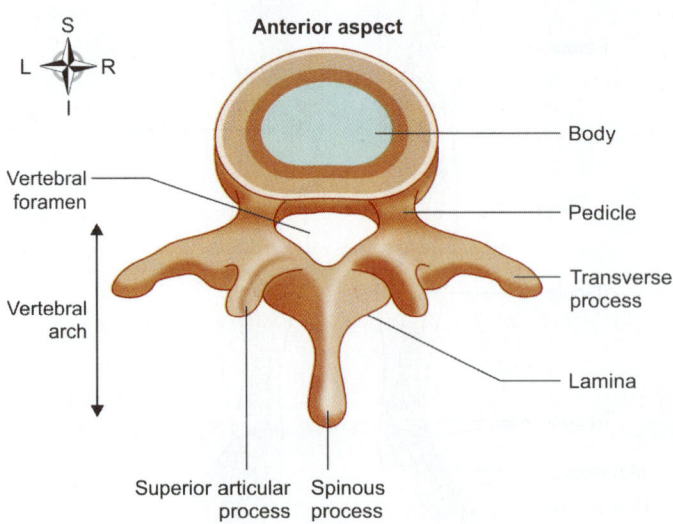

Fig. 6.2: Lumbar vertebra

Sternum and Ribs

- Sternum is a flat narrow bone located in the middle of the front part of the chest.
- There are twelve pairs of ribs. Posteriorly, ribs are connected to thoracic vertebrae and anteriorly to the sternum. Lower two ribs are not attached to the sternum and are called floating ribs.
- Thoracic vertebrae, sternum and ribs together form the thoracic cage.

Appendicular Skeleton

Appendicular skeleton consists of (Fig. 6.3):
- Shoulder girdle with upper limb, and
- Pelvic girdle with lower limb.

Shoulder Girdle and Upper Limb

- Shoulder girdle consists of two clavicles and two scapulae.
- The clavicle is an 's' shaped long bone. Medially, it joins with sternum and forms sternoclavicular joint. Laterally, it forms acromioclavicular joint with acromion process of scapula.
- Lateral angle of the scapula has a shallow articular surface called the glenoid cavity. It articulates with the head of the humerus and forms shoulder joint.
- Humerus is the long bone of the upper arm. Upper end has a round smooth head. Lower end is articulated with radius and ulna and forms elbow joint.
- There are two bones of forearm—radius and ulna. Ulna is longer than the radius and located medial to the radius.
- There are eight irregular small bones called carpal bones. They are arranged in two rows and form wrist.
- Metacarpals form the palm of the hand. They are five in number.
- Phalanges form the fingers of the hand. They are 14 in number—three for each finger and two for thumb.

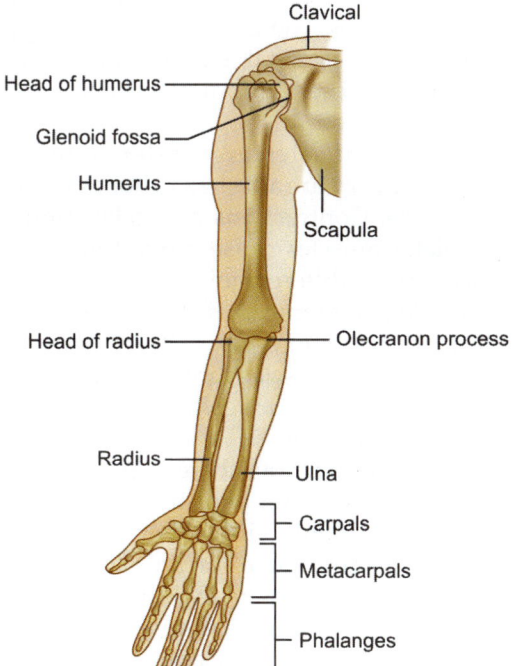
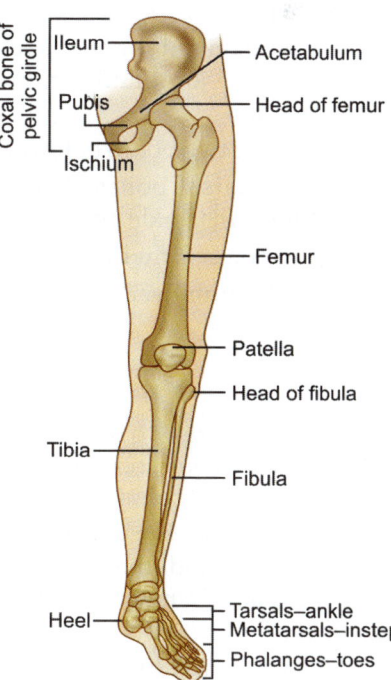

Fig. 6.3: Shoulder girdle and pelvic girdle

Pelvic Girdle and Lower Limb

- Pelvic girdles consist of two innominate bones—one on either sides of sacrum and coccyx.
- Sacrum and coccyx form the centre back part of pelvic girdle.
- Innominate bones or hip bones are made by fusion of three bones—ilium, ischium and pubis.
- There is depression on the hip bone called accetabulum. This articulates with the head of the femur bone and constitutes hip joint.
- Innominate or hip bones join together anteriorly at midline, and form pubic symphysis.
- Bones of the lower limb are femur, tibia, fibula, patella, tarsal bones, metatarsals and phalanges.
- Femur or thigh bone is the longest and strongest bone of the human body. Above, it joins with the accetabulum and forms hip joint. Below, it articulates with tibia and forms the knee joint.
- Patella is a round, circular bone, situated in front of the knee joint and commonly known as knee cap.
- Tibia and fibula are two bones of lower leg.
- There are seven tarsal bones. They join together and form the ankle and heel.
- Five metatarsal bones form instep.
- Phalanges are 14 in number. They are bones of the toes.

JOINTS

- A joint is the site where two or more bones articulate or join together. It can be a fibrous joint, cartilaginous joint or synovial joint.
- In fibrous joints, bones are articulated by tough fibrous tissue and, therefore, movement is not possible. *Example:* Joint between the skull bones.
- When bones are joined by white fibrous cartilage, it is called cartilaginous joint. Limited movement is possible in this type of Joint. *Example*: Joint between the vertebrae.
- Synovial joints are freely movable joints. Articular surface of bones is covered by hyaline cartilage. The joints are surrounded by a fibrous capsule that holds the bones together. Inner surface of the joint is covered by a synovial membrane which secretes synovial fluid to lubricate the joint.

Types of Synovial Joint

- **Ball and socket joint:** Shoulder and hip joints
- **Hinge joint:** Knee, elbow and finger joints
- **Pivot joint:** Between the atlas and axis vertebrae
- **Gliding joint:** Between tarsal bones and carpal bones
- **Ellipsoid joint:** Joint between metacarpals, metatarsals and phalanges.

SKELETAL MUSCLES

- Muscles are made up of highly specialized thin, elongated contractile cells called muscle fibres. There are three distinct types of muscle—skeletal, smooth and cardiac. Smooth and cardiac muscles are not under voluntary control.
- Skeletal muscles are under voluntary control. They are attached to bones via their tendons. Contractions and relaxations of skeletal muscles cause movements of the skeleton at different joints.
- Muscle cells or muscle fibres are responsible for contractions and relaxations. Contractility of muscle fibres is governed by protein filaments myosin and actin present in the cytoplasm.
- During contraction, there is no change in the length of actin and myosin filaments. Actin filaments slide over the myosin filaments and move inwards towards the centre of a sarcomere and thus reduce the total length of muscle fibres.
- During relaxation, actin and myosin occupy their normal position and muscle fibres resume their normal length.

- Muscle fibres contract in response to stimulation from nerve fibre. Axons of motor neurons carry impulses to skeletal muscle and stimulate to contract. Stimulation of motor neuron releases the neurotransmitter acetylcholine (ACh). Acetylcholine diffuses across the synaptic cleft and acts on motor end plate and causes contractions of the muscle cell.

DISEASES OF MUSCULOSKELETAL SYSTEM

Arthritis: Arthritis means inflammation of the joints. Rheumatoid arthritis, osteoarthritis and gouty arthritis are some of the common arthritis.

Osteoporosis: It is the condition characterized by reduced bone density. Common features of osteoporosis are:

- Skeletal deformity
- Bone pain
- Fractures of hip, wrist and vertebra.

Osteomyelitis: This is a bacterial infection of bone usually after open fracture or bony surgical procedures.

Myasthenia gravis: This is an autoimmune disease characterized by progressive and extensive muscle weakness. Eyelid muscles are affected first and cause ptosis. This is followed by neck and limb muscles weakness.

CHAPTER 7

The Nervous System

The nervous system receives, detects and responds to changes inside and outside the body. The nervous system consists of the brain, spinal cord and peripheral nerves.

Major Functions of Nervous System

- To control and coordinate various voluntary and involuntary activities of the body.
- To regulate internal environment of the body.
- To react according to changes in the external environment.
- To remember, think and reason out of an incidence.

Parts of the Nervous System

- The nervous system consists of two parts—central nervous system and peripheral nervous system.
- Central nervous system consists of:
  - Brain
  - Spinal cord
- Peripheral nervous system consists of:
  - Cranial nerves
  - Spinal nerves

CENTRAL NERVOUS SYSTEM

Central nervous system or brain and spinal cord are enclosed and protected within the skull and vertebral column. The brain and spinal cord are covered by three layers of meninges (membranous structure). They are dura mater, arachnoid mater and pia mater. Arachnoid and pia maters are separated by subarachnoid space, which contains cerebrospinal fluid (CSF).

Cerebrospinal fluid

It is a clear slightly alkaline fluid with a specific gravity of 1.005. It consists of water, mineral salts, glucose and small amounts of plasma proteins, creatinine and urea. Volume of CSF is about 150 ml in adult and maintains pressure approximately 10 cm H_2O. It is secreted at a rate of 0.5 ml by choroid plexus of lateral ventricles.

Cerebrospinal fluid acts as a cushion between the brain and skull. It keeps the brain and spinal cord moist and exchanges the nutrients and waste products from the central nervous system.

Brain

It consists of the following parts (Fig. 7.1):
- Cerebrum
- Thalamus

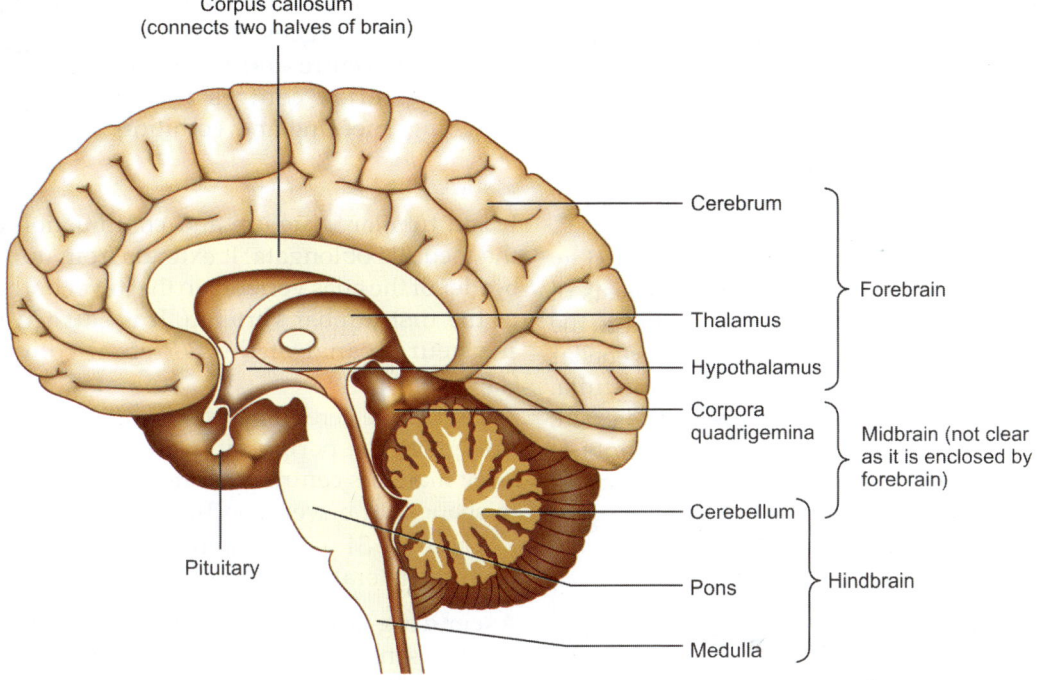

Fig. 7.1: Brain in vertical section

- Hypothalamus
- Midbrain
- Cerebellum
- Pons
- Medulla oblongata

Cerebrum

- It is the largest part of the brain, consists of two cerebral hemispheres joined together by a broad thick band called corpus callosum.
- Each cerebral hemisphere is divided into four lobes—frontal, parietal, temporal and occipital. Cerebral cortex has many in-folding or convolutions called gyri.
- Outer region of the cerebral hemisphere is grey in colour and packed with nerve cells called cerebral cortex. Inner white matter of cerebrum contains axons which connect various parts of the brain.

- Cerebral cortex consists of three areas:
  a. Sensory receives sensations from receptors.
  b. Motor transmits impulses to various organs and controls voluntary movements.
  c. Association area is associated with memory, learning, reasoning and intelligence.

Thalamus

It is present in the centre of the forebrain. All sensory impulses pass through the thalamus. It interprets them and then sends them to an appropriate region of the cerebral cortex.

Hypothalamus

It is present beneath the thalamus. It co-ordinates various autonomous activities of the body including water balance. It controls the secretion of hormones from the anterior and posterior pituitary glands.

Midbrain

Midbrain connects the forebrain and hind-brain. It has four quadrigemina which are reflex centres for eye movement and auditory responses. Lower parts are associated with motor reflexes and balance reflexes.

Cerebellum

It is situated in posterior cranial fossa below the posterior part of cerebrum. It consists of two cerebellar hemispheres and similar to the cerebrum, it also has an outer grey cerebellar cortex and inner white cerebellar medulla. Cerebellum is the motor centre of the brain, concerned with coordinating movements of skeletal muscles, maintenance of posture or equilibrium.

Pons

It acts as a bridge carrying ascending and descending tracts between the brain and spinal cord.

Medulla Oblongata

It is the lowest part of the brain located at the base of the skull. Below it continues as spinal cord. Posterior medulla controls the activities of the internal organs. It has a cardiac centre, respiratory centre and vasomotor centre. It also has reflex centres for swallowing, coughing, sneezing and vomiting.

Spinal Cord

It is a tubular structure and continuation of the medulla oblongata. It extends from upper border of the atlas vertebra to the lower border of the first lumbar vertebra. It is situated in the neural canal of the vertebral column (Fig. 7.2).

Unlike the cerebral cortex, white matter is present at the periphery in the spinal cord. Grey matter is centrally located and butterfly in shape in transverse section.

There are 31 pairs of spinal nerves emerges from the lateral side of the spinal cord.

Ascending tract: Ascending nerve tracts conduct sensory impulses from the spinal cord to the brain.

Descending tract: Descending nerve tracts conduct motor information from the brain to the spinal cord.

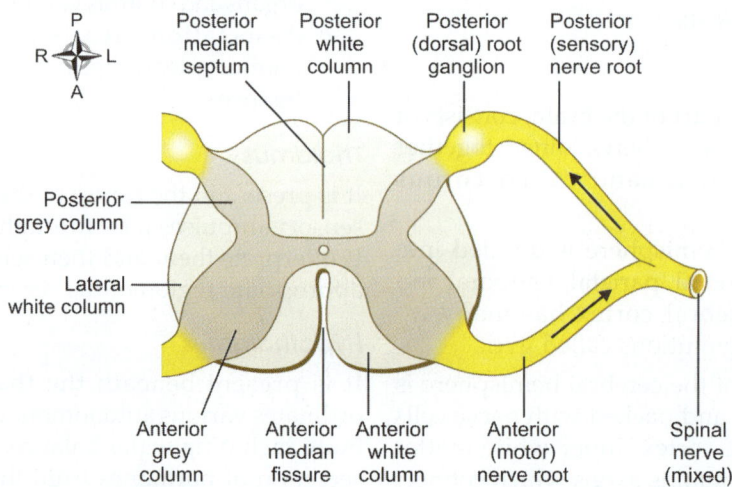

Fig. 7.2: Transverse section of the spinal cord

PERIPHERAL NERVOUS SYSTEM

Peripheral nervous system (PNS) consists of two types of nerves:

- Spinal nerves arise from the spinal cord.
- Cranial nerves arise from the brain.

Spinal Nerves

- There are 31 pairs of spinal nerves originate from the spinal cord.
    - I. Cervical nerves—8 pairs
    - II. Thoracic nerves—12 pairs
    - III. Lumbar nerves—5 pairs
    - IV. Sacral nerves—5 pairs
    - V. Coccygeal nerves—1 pair
- All spinal nerves are mixed nerves contain sensory and motor neurons. Spinal nerve is attached to the spinal cord by dorsal root carrying sensory neurons and ventral root carrying motor neurons.
- Dorsal root of spinal cord carries impulses from receptor to the spinal cord while ventral root carries impulses from the spinal cord to muscles.
- Spinal cord is the centre of reflex arcs.

Cranial Nerves

- There are 12 pairs of cranial nerves arising from nuclei situated at the inferior surface of the brain.
- Cranial nerve could be sensory, motor or mixed.
    - I. Olfactory nerve (sensory)
    - II. Optic nerve (sensory)
    - III. Oculomotor nerve (motor)
    - IV. Trochlear nerve (motor)
    - V. Trigeminal nerve (mixed)
    - VI. Abducens nerve (motor)
    - VII. Facial nerves (mixed)
    - VIII. Vestibulocochlear nerve (sensory)
    - IX. Glossopharyngeal nerve (mixed)
    - X. Vagus nerve (mixed)
    - XI. Accessory nerve (motor)
    - XII. Hypoglossal nerve (motor)

AUTONOMIC NERVOUS SYSTEM

- Autonomic nervous system controls the involuntary functions of visceral organs like heart, lungs, kidney and gastrointestinal tract.
- Autonomic nervous system consists of three important structures.
    - a. *Preganglionic fibres*: They are motor neurons, emerge from the central nervous system and end at autonomic ganglion.
    - b. *Autonomic ganglia*: They are bulbous structure. Here preganglionic fibres synapse with cells of postganglionic fibres.
    - c. *Postganglionic fibres*: They start from autonomic ganglia and end at targeted organs.
- Autonomic nervous system consists of the the parasympathetic and sympathetic system. Every organ has parasympathetic as well as sympathetic nerve. They have usually opposite effects.

SENSORY ORGANS

The Eye (Fig. 7.3)

It is the sensory organ of sight. It is a spherical structure of about 2.5 cm in diameter. It is situated in the orbital cavity and supplied by the optic nerve.

There are three layers of tissue, constitutes the wall of the eye.

1. Outer fibrous layer—sclera and cornea
2. Middle vascular layer—choroid, ciliary body, iris and lens.
3. Inner nervous tissue layer—retina

Sclera

- It is a white opaque fibroelastic capsule.
- It maintains the shape of the eyeball and protects the inner layers of the eye.
- Eye muscles are attached to the sclera and are responsible for the movements of the eyeball.

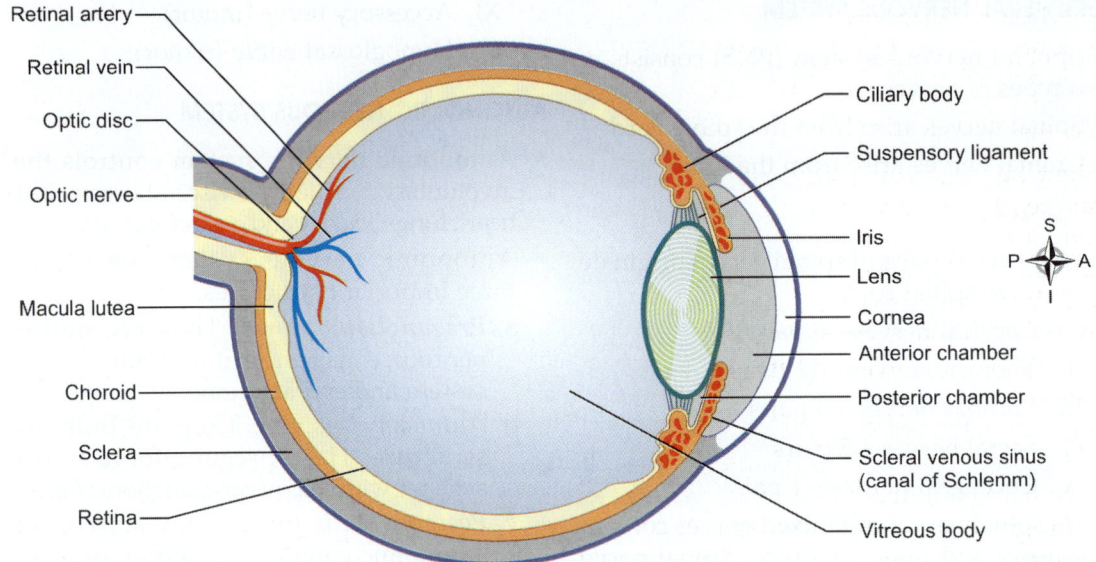

Fig. 7.3: Vertical section of the eye

Cornea

- It is a thin transparent front part of the sclera.
- Light rays pass through the cornea to reach the retina.
- It is convex anteriorly and involves in the refraction of light rays to focus them on the retina.
- Conjunctiva is a thin transparent layer which protects the cornea.

Choroid

- It is highly pigmented middle layer of the eyeball. It prevents reflection of light within the eye.
- It is very rich in blood vessels and provides nutrition to the retina.

Ciliary Body

- It is the anterior continuation of the choroid and consists of ciliary muscles.
- The lens is attached to the ciliary body by suspensory ligaments. Contractions and relaxations of the ciliary muscle fibres control the size and thickness of the lens.

Iris

It is a pigmented circle of the muscular diaphragm in front of the lens. It controls the size of the pupil and amount of light entering into the eye.

Lens

It is a transparent biconvex body located immediately behind the pupil. Contraction and relaxation of ciliary muscles change the shape of the lens for viewing the objects at different distances.

Retina

- It is the inner most layer of the eyeball and consists of two types of photoreceptor cells called rods and cones.
- It also contains bipolar nerve cells, retinal ganglia and horizontal and amacrine cells.
- An inverted image of the object is formed at the retina.
- Optic nerve: It is the second cranial nerve and carries sensory impulses from retina to the cerebral cortex.

- Blind spot: It is the area of the retina from where the optic nerve leaves the eyeball. It is not sensitive to light and, therefore, image is not formed at the blind spot.

Mechanism of Vision

Light rays from an object enter into the eye and reach the retina through cornea, aqueous humour, lens and vitreous humour. Light rays are converged by curvature of cornea and lens and finally focus on the retina to form an inverted image. According to the distance of an object from the eye, lens changes its convexity, changes refractive power and thus focuses on the retina.

Normal eye is able to accommodate light from objects from 25 cm to infinity.

Image at the retina is inverted which is reversed by the brain to form image at right direction.

The Ear

Ear is the organ of hearing and balance. It is supplied by the 8th cranial nerve (vesti-bulocochlear). Cochlear part of the vesti-bulocochlear nerve is concerned with hearing and vestibular part with balance.

The ear consists of three main parts—air-filled external ear and middle ear and fluid-filled inner ear (Fig. 7.4).

External Ear

- It consists of ear lobe or pinna, auditory canal and tympanic membrane.
- Tympanic membrane is a thin tight membrane lies between the external ear and middle ear. Sound waves strike on the tympanic membrane and produce vibrations.

Middle Ear

- Middle ear consists of three bony ossicles—malleus, incus and stapes. One end of malleus is attached to the inner surface of the tympanic membrane and an other end is connected to incus which is in turn, joined to stapes. Stapes is connected to a membranous structure called oval window, which leads to inner ear.

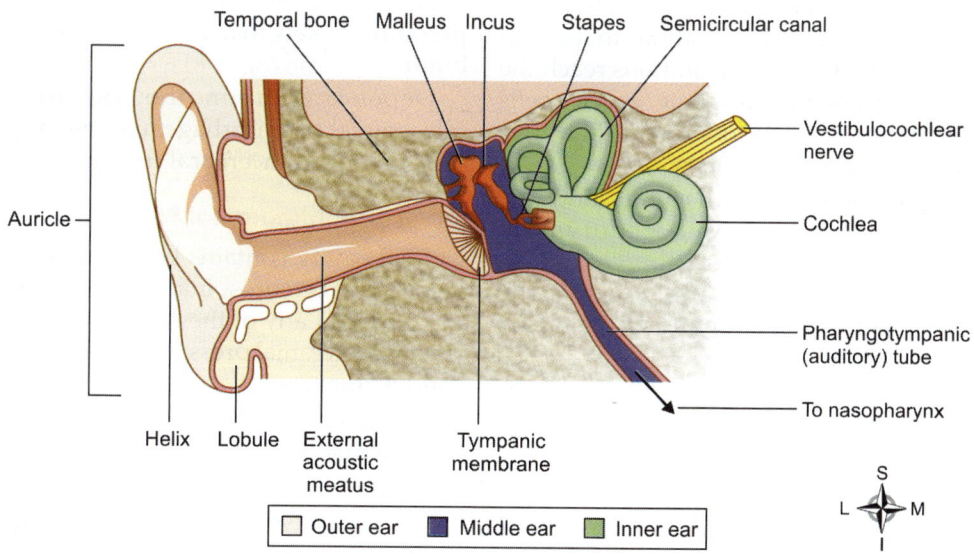

Fig. 7.4: Structure and function of the ear

- Middle ear opens into pharynx through the Eustachian tube.

Inner Ear

- Inner ear consists of cochlea, semicircular canals and vestibule. Cochlea is a spiral-shaped structure. Inner cavity of the cochlea is divided by membranous structure and forms three parallel tubes.
- The middle canal of cochlea contains 'organ of Corti' or receptor hair cells which transform sound vibrations to nerve impulses. Semicircular canals are a set of three canals arranged at right angles to each other. They contain sensory cells for maintenance of body position (dynamic equilibrium).
- Vestibule joins the base of the semicircular canal to the cochlea. It is concerned with static equilibrium.

Mechanism of Hearing and Balance

- Sound waves enter through the auditory canal and produce vibrations on the tympanic membrane. Tympanic membrane transmits the vibration to three bony ossicles of middle ear. Stapes magnifies vibration by lever like action of other two ossicles and transmits vibrations to the oval window. Finally, these vibrations reach the cochlear canals and stimulate sensory cells to the organ of Corti to transmit impulses to the brain via the auditory nerve.
- The three semicircular canals and the vestibule are filled with endolymph. Endolymph moves with the change in position of the body and touches the sensory hair to send stimulus to brain for maintaining balance.

COMMON DISORDERS OF THE NERVOUS SYSTEM

Head Injury

Head injury is one of the most serious outcomes of an accident. Significant damage of brain may occur even in absence of any apparent injury on the head, face or skull. At the site of injury, there may be a scalp wound, depressed skull fracture, black eye or bleeding from ear and nose.

Mechanism of Head Injury

Normally brain floats relatively freely in a cushion of CSF. Impact on the skull produces sudden movement of the brain within the skull, causes acceleration-deceleration brain injuries. Nerve cells may be damaged due to movement of the brain over the rough surface of bone especially at the base of the skull. Nerve fibres may be damaged due to stretching. Rupture of blood vessels cause haemorrhage and raised intracranial pressure.

If a person survives following injury, complications may occur during the next 48–72 hours. Complications are raised intracranial pressure, infections and further secondary brain damage.

Intracranial Haemorrhage

Intracranial haemorrhage may cause secondary brain damage at the site of injury, on the opposite side of the brain or diffuse brain injury. If bleeding continues, intracranial pressure is likely to increase and compress the brain.

Depending upon the site of injury, intracranial haemorrhage may be extradural, subdural or intracerebral in origin.

Increased Intracranial Pressure

Cranial cavity contains brain, cerebral blood vessels and cerebrospinal fluid (CSF). Increase in volume of any of these components causes rise in intracranial pressure because it is a rigid compartment.

Therefore, the rise in intracranial pressure may be due to the following reasons:

- Cerebral oedema
- Increased volume of cerebrospinal fluid (hydrocephalus)

- Intracranial space-occupying lesions
  - Haemorrhage or haematoma (traumatic or spontaneous)
  - Intracranial tumour

Increased intracranial pressure is associated with bradycardia and hypertension. Further rise in ICP reduces cerebral blood flow, cerebral hypoxia, hypercarbia and brain damage.

Severe rise in intracranial pressure causes displacement of the brain, herniation, compression of vital centre and death.

CHAPTER 8

The Endocrine System

Endocrine system consists of endocrine glands, located at different parts of the body. Endocrine glands are ductless glands and consist of groups of secretory cells surrounded by the capillary network. Secretory cells secrete hormone directly into the bloodstream to reach target tissues or organs.

The principal endocrinal glands are:

- Pituitary
- Adrenal
- Thyroid
- Parathyroid
- Pancreas
- Thymus
- Pineal
- Testes
- Ovaries

PITUITARY GLAND

- Pituitary gland is a small pea-shaped gland, weight is about 500 mg and is located at the hypophyseal fossa of the sphenoid bone below the hypothalamus.
- Pituitary gland works under the influence of hypothalamus and it influences almost all the endocrine glands of the body. So it is called master gland.

- Pituitary gland consists of three lobes—anterior lobe, intermediate lobe and posterior lobe.
- **Anterior pituitary:** It secretes six main hormones.
  - Thyroid-stimulating hormone (TSH) stimulates thyroid to produce thyroxine.
  - Adrenocorticotropic hormone (ACTH) stimulates the adrenal cortex to produce corticosteroid hormones.
  - Follicle-stimulating hormone (FSH) stimulates ovarian follicles of ovaries in female and seminiferous tubules of testes in the male.
  - Luteinizing hormone (LH) stimulates corpus luteum to produce progesterone in females and interstitial cells of testes to produce testosterone in males.
  - Growth hormone (GH) stimulates body growth by stimulating cell mitosis and protein synthesis.
  - Prolactin or luteotrophic hormone (LTH) controls growth of breast tissue and secretion of milk.

First four hormones act on other endocrine glands and controles the secretion of hormones from target glands. They are collectively known as tropic hormones.

- **Intermediate pituitary:** It secretes melano-cytes-stimulating hormone (MSH) which stimulates the formation of melanin (black pigments).
- **Posterior pituitary:** It secretes two hormones.
  - *Vasopressin or antidiuretic hormone (ADH):* It is a water-retaining hormone and reduces the volume of urine. It is also a vasoconstrictor and increases arterial blood pressure.
  - *Oxytocin:* It causes contractions of uterine smooth muscles during parturition. It also contracts mammary gland muscles and helps in the ejection of milk during breastfeeding.

ADRENAL GLANDS

Two small yellowish glands are situated just above the kidney and hence also known as suprarenal glands. Each adrenal gland consists of two parts—external adrenal cortex and internal adrenal medulla.

Adrenal Cortex

Hormones produced by the adrenal cortex are called corticoids or cortical steroids. There are three types of cortical steroids.

- **Mineralocorticoids:** Aldosterone is the main mineralocorticosteroid. It helps to maintain water and electrolyte balance. Main role of aldosterone is:
  - To stimulate kidney to reabsorb sodium and thus maintain sodium level and blood volume, and
  - To stimulate kidney to excrete potassium.
- **Glucocorticoids:** They are responsible for the breakdown of protein and fat into glucose. They raise blood sugar level and help the body to recover from stress.
- **Gonadocorticoids:** They are sex corticoids but play a minor role as quantity is very less.

Adrenal Medulla

Hormones secreted by the adrenal medulla are adrenaline and noradrenaline. Effects of these hormones are similar to those produced by stimulation of the sympathetic nervous system. They are called emergency hormone or hormone of the fight.

THYROID GLAND

- It is situated in front of larynx and trachea. It consists of two lobes joined by a narrow isthmus and looks like a butterfly.
- Thyroid gland produces three hormones.
  - Thyroxine or T_4
  - Triiodothyronine or T_3
  - Calcitonin
- Thyroxine (T_4) and triiodothyronine (T_3) control the rate of cellular metabolism. They increase the basal metabolic rate and heat production. They also regulate the metabolism of carbohydrates, proteins and fats.
- Calcitonin inhibits the calcium loss in bones. It regulates the plasma calcium level of blood.

PANCREAS

Pancreas is an exocrine as well as an endocrine gland. Clusters of cells called 'islets of Langerhans' secrete hormones.

It consists of three types of cells—α cells produce glucagon, β cells produce insulin and δ cells produce somatostatin.

Insulin and glucagon have antagonistic effects on the metabolism of carbohydrates and fats.

DISORDERS OF ENDOCRINE GLAND

Piluitary Gland

- *Gigantism and acromegaly* are due to hyper-secretion of growth hormone.
- *Hyperprolactinaemia* is due to hypersecretion of prolactin. It causes galactorrhoea, amenorrhoea and sterility.

- *Pituitary dwarfism* is due to severe deficiency of growth hormone. It causes small stature but normally proportioned. Cognitive development is also not affected.
- *Diabetes incipidus* is a disorder of posterior pituitary. It is caused by hyposecretion of ADH due to damage of the hypothalamus. Water reabsorption by renal tubules is grossly impaired, leading to excretion of the large amount of diluted urine.

Adrenal Gland

- *Addison's disease* is due to destruction of the adrenal cortex, leading to chronic adrenocortical insufficiency. There are hyposecretions of glucocorticoid and mineralocorticoid hormones. It is characterized by muscle weakness and wasting, and gastrointestinal disturbances.
- *Cushing syndrome* is due to hypersecretion of glucocorticoid by adrenal cortex. It is characterized by abdominal obesity with a wasting of limb muscles, hyperglycaemia, hypernatraemia, hypokalaemia and hypertension.
- Aldosteronism is due to excessive secretion of mineralocorticoids specially aldosteron. It is characterized by hypernatraemia, hypokalaemia, hypertension and increased blood volume.
- *Pheochromocytoma* is a hormone-secreting tumour of the adrenal medulla. It causes excessive secretion of adrenaline and noradrenaline. It is characterized by hypertension, weight loss, excessive sweating, nervousness and anxiety.

Thyroid Gland

- *Hypothyroidism* is due to deficiency of thyroid hormone T_3 and T_4. It causes slowing of metabolic rate, decreased heart rate, decreased respiratory rate and sluggish reflexes. Basal metabolic rate is reduced by 20–30%. It causes physical and mental retardation. It produces cretinism in children and myxedema in adults.
- *Hyperthyroidism* is due to overactivity of the thyroid gland and excessive secretion of thyroid hormones. It is characterized by increased metabolic rate, increased respiratory rate and raised temperature. It causes nervousness and irritability.

Pancreas

Diabetes mellitus is caused by under activity of β cells of the pancreas leading to a deficiency of insulin. It is characterized by hyperglycaemia and glycosuria. There is breakdown of fat and protein and conversion into glucose. Increased oxidation of fat produces increased ketone body and blood cholesterol level. Long-term diabetes mellitus produces end-organ damage due to macrovascular and microvascular involvement.

CHAPTER 9

The Reproductive System

Reproduction is the process of producing young ones of its own kind by an organism. This is one of the properties of the living organisms. Human reproduces by sexual reproduction. Female sex cell, ovum fuses with the male gamete, sperm by the process of fertilization and zygote is formed. Zygote develops into a new individual.

Testes and ovaries are the primary male and female reproductive organs which produce sperms and eggs, respectively.

MALE REPRODUCTIVE SYSTEM

Male reproductive system (Fig. 9.1) consists of:
- Testes,
- Sperm ducts,
- Accessory glands, and
- Penis.

Testes

- Two testes are suspended in thin pouches of skin and connective tissue called scrotal sacs, present outside the abdominal cavity and just behind the penis.
- Testes are 4–5 cm long, 2.5 cm wide and 3 cm thick, oval, soft, pinkish structure.
- Testes are consisting of seminiferous tubules which take part in spermatogenesis and produce spermatids.

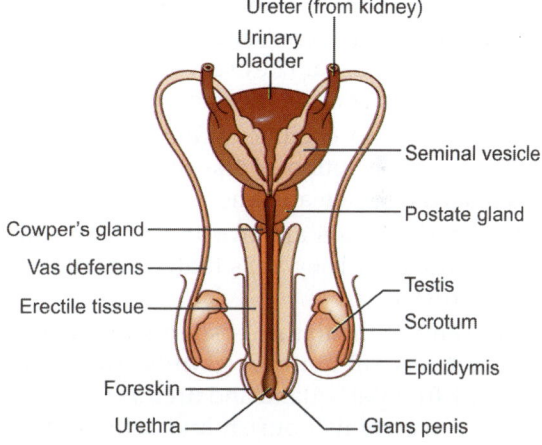

Fig. 9.1: Male reproductive system

- Small group of cells called interstitial cells are present in between the seminiferous tubules. Interstitial cells secrete male sex hormone, testosterone.
- Testosterone is responsible for the development of sex organs, secondary sexual character and maintenance of spermatogenesis.

Sperm Ducts

- Small tiny ductules from seminiferous tubules unite and form vasa efferentia. They conduct spermatids into the epididymis.

Maturation of spermatids takes place and finally store as spermatozoa in the epididymis.

- Sperm duct originates from the epididymus and carries spermatozoa. Sperm duct joins with the duct of seminal vesicles to form ejaculatory duct.
- Ejaculatory duct passes through the prostate gland and opens into the urethra. Ducts from Cowper's gland also open directly into the urethra before it enters the penis.

Accessory Glands

- Male accessory glands include two seminal vesicles, prostate gland and two Cowper's glands.
- Seminal vesicles are situated between urinary bladder and rectum. Secretions of seminal vesicles carry via a duct and mixed with spermatozoa. They serve as a medium for transportation of the sperm.
- Prostate gland encircles urethra closed to its origin. Secretion of the prostate gland makes the semen alkaline.
- Cowper's glands are two in number and oval in shape. They are situated just below the prostate.

  The semen is a mixture of spermatozoa and secretions of seminal glands, prostate gland, Cowper's gland and urethral glands. These secretions nourish and activate the spermatozoa to swim. Semen contains citrate, ascorbic acid, acid phosphatase, fructose and hormone like prostaglandin.

Penis

- Penis is an ejaculatory organ, situated in front of the scrotum. It is used for expelling semen and urine.
- During sexual stimulation, large amount of blood flows into the penis and makes it rigid and erect.
- During ejaculation, the sphincter at the base of the urinary bladder is closed and thus only semen is ejaculated.

FEMALE REPRODUCTIVE SYSTEM

The female reproductive system consists of two ovaries, two fallopian tubes, uterus, vagina, accessory genital glands and mammary glands (Fig. 9.2).

Ovaries

- They are oval-shaped structures, attached to the posterior abdominal wall by meso-ovarian. Ovary produces ova or eggs. Usually, the one egg matures in each ovary in every alternative month. Every month ovum is released by the rupture of follicles which is called ovulation.
- After ovulation, the remaining part of the follicle is called corpus luteum. Oestrogen is secreted by corpus luteum.

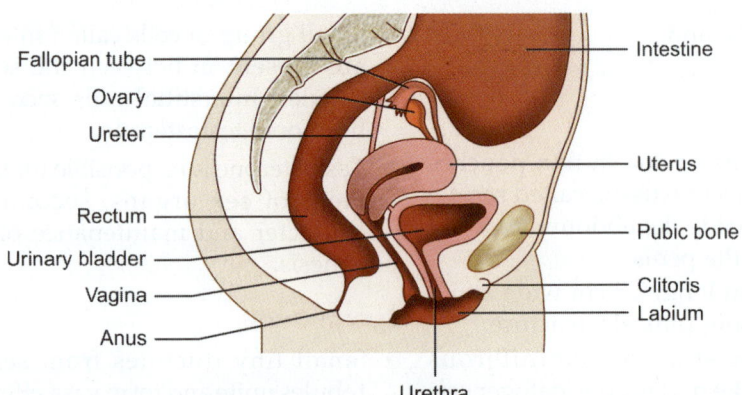

Fallopian tube — Ovary — Ureter — Rectum — Urinary bladder — Vagina — Anus — Intestine — Uterus — Pubic bone — Clitoris — Labium — Urethra

Fig. 9.2: Female reproductive system

Fallopian Tubes

- They are 10 to 12 cm long muscular tubes, located on either side of uterus.
- Each fallopian tube consists of broad funnel-shaped infundibulum, long thin-walled tubular structure ampulla, thick short isthmus and uterine part of tube.
- It carries ovum from the ovary to the uterus and provides the optimum environment for fertilization.

Uterus

- The uterus is the pear-shaped, hollow muscular structure situated between the urinary bladder and the rectum.
- Uterus has three parts—fundus, body or isthmus and cervix.
- Uterus consists of three layers—outer perimetrium, middle muscular layer myometrium and inner mucous membrane endometrium. Endometrium undergoes cyclic changes during different phases of the menstrual cycle.
- Uterus receives fertilized ovum and offers the proper environment for the growth of the fetus.

Vagina

The vagina is a large muscular tube of about 7.5 cm long. Above it is continued as cervical part of the uterus. Below it opens in the external female genitalia called vulva.

Bartholin's Gland

Two Bartholin's glands are located on either side of the vaginal orifice. They secrete clear fluid which serves as a lubricant.

SEX HORMONES

There are mainly three types of hormones. Oestrogen and progesterone are secreted in females. Testosterone is secreted in males.

CHAPTER 10

The Urinary System

The urinary system is the main excretory system of human body. It consists of:
- Two kidneys
- Two ureters
- One urinary bladder
- One urethra

KIDNEYS

Kidneys are bean-shaped reddish brown and slightly flattened organ. Each adult kidney is about 10–12 cm long, 5–7 cm wide and 2–3 cm in thickness. Weight of each kidney is approximately 135 to 150 grams.

These kidneys are located on the posterior abdominal wall behind the peritoneum on each side of vertebral column. They are situated at the level of 12th thoracic vertebra to the 3rd lumbar vertebra. The left kidney is slightly above the right kidney.

On the medial side of kidney at the centre, there is a notch called hilum from where renal arteries, vein and ureter enter.

Organs Associated with the Kidney

Right Kidney

- Superiorly—right adrenal gland
- Posteriorly—diaphragm and posterior abdominal muscles
- Anteriorly—right lobe of the liver, duodenum and hepatic flexure of the colon

Left Kidney

- Superiorly—left adrenal gland
- Posteriorly—diaphragm and posterior abdominal muscles
- Anteriorly—spleen, pancreas, stomach, jejunum and splenic flexure of colon

URETER

Each kidney has one ureter which carries urine from kidney to the bladder. It is about 25 to 30 cm long and 3 mm in diameter. It opens in the posterior surface of the bladder.

URINARY BLADDER

Urinary bladder is a reservoir for urine. It continuously receives urine from kidney and intermittently as well as voluntarily evacuated through urethral orifice. It is pear-shaped and situated in the pelvic cavity.

There are three orifices in the bladder wall form a triangle or trigone. Upper two orifices on the posterior wall are ureteric opening and lower orifice located at the neck of the bladder is the opening of the urethra.

URETHRA

It is a canal extending from the neck of the bladder to the external urethral orifice. It is longer in the male than female. It has two sphincters. The internal urethral sphincter controls the outflow of urine from the bladder. External urethral sphincter is located at the external urethral orifice, which is under voluntary control.

GROSS ANATOMY OF THE KIDNEY

Three distinct areas can be identified in a longitudinal section of the kidney.

- Outer most fibrous capsule
- Immediately below the capsule, a layer of reddish-brown tissue is called cortex
- Inner most layer consists of the pale conical-shaped renal pyramid is called medulla (Fig. 10.1).

The urine produced in the kidney passes through renal papilla → minor calyx → major calyx and finally reaches to the renal pelvis.

MICROSCOPIC STRUCTURE OF THE KIDNEY

The Nephron

Each kidney contains about 1 million functional units; known as nephron. Each nephron consists of 5 parts (Fig. 10.2):
1. Renal corpuscle
   a. Bowman's capsule
   b. Glomerulus
2. Proximal convoluted tubule
3. Loop of Henle
   a. Descending limb
   b. Ascending limb
4. Distal convoluted tubule
5. Collecting tubule

Bowman's Capsule

It is a cup-shaped hollow structure, lined by two epithelial layers. It encloses a network of capillaries called glomerulus.

Glomerulus

It is a network of capillaries receives blood from renal artery through afferent arteriole.

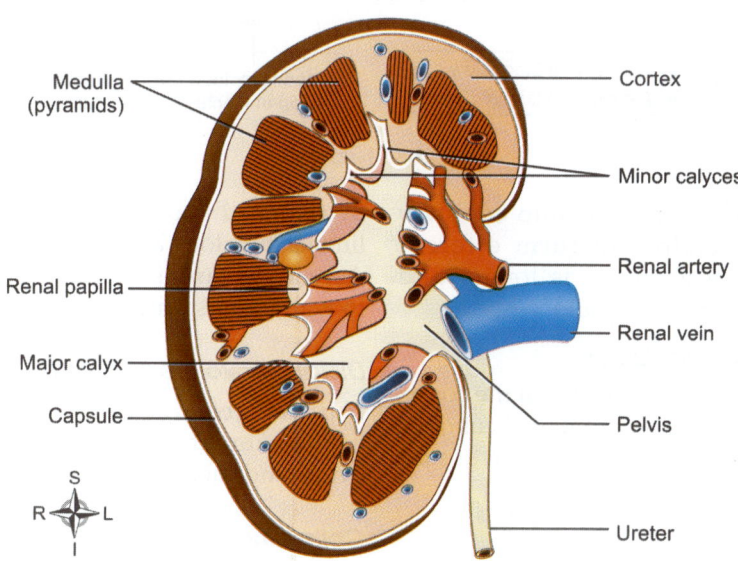

Fig. 10.1: Longitudinal section of kidney

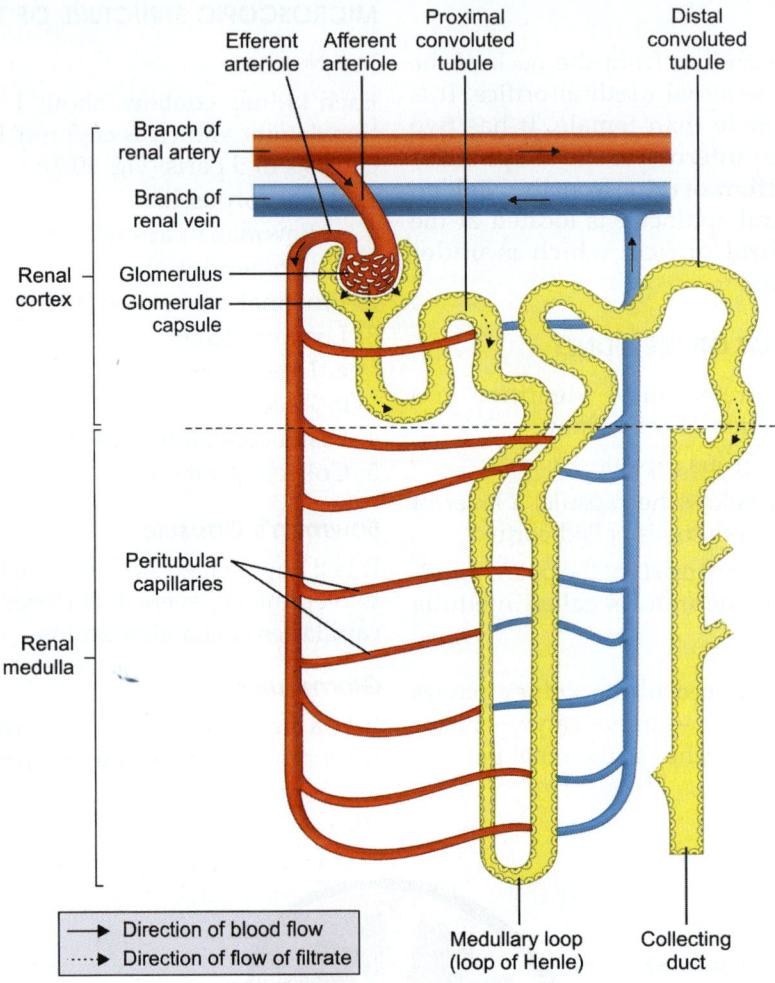

Fig. 10.2: Nephron

Afferent arteriole breaks up into capillary networks that rejoin and form efferent arteriole. Efferent arteriole is longer and narrower than afferent arteriole.

Proximal Convoluted Tubule

It is the first coiled tubule located at the cortex region of kidney. It is lined by ciliated cuboidal epithelium. It allows the reabsorption of salts by active absorption.

Loop of Henle

It is U shaped loop located partially at cortical and partially at medullary region. It is lined

by flattened cuboid epithelium. Descending limb is thin, long and free permeable to water. Ascending limb is thicker and impermeable to water and sodium chloride.

Distal Convoluted Tubule

It is the second coiled tube responsible for active tubular secretions of selective ions, drugs and metabolic waste.

Collecting Tubule

Collecting tubule collects urine produced by proximal parts of the nephron. Many collecting tubules join and form collecting duct, which ultimately opens into the renal pelvis.

FORMATION OF URINE

There are three processes involved in the formation of urine.
- Filtration
- Selective reabsorption
- Active tubular secretion

Glomerular Filtration

Blood of the glomerulus capillaries is filtered and protein-free glomerular filtrate is collected in Bowman's capsule. Glomerular filtrate is actually filtered blood without blood cells and plasma proteins.

Glomerular filtration is a physical process determined by the hydrostatic pressure of the blood.

Net filtration pressure = Hydrostatic pressure of glomerular capillaries – (osmotic pressure of plasma proteins + glomerular filtration pressure)

So, fall in hydrostatic pressure or blood pressure reduces filtration rate. Normal glomerular filtration rate (GFR) is 125 ml/min.

Regulation of Glomerular Filtration

Glomerular filtration is regulated automatically by two mechanisms.

a. **Myogenic mechanism:** Normally rise in blood pressure should stretch the afferent arteriole and should increase blood flow as well as glomerular filtration. But the stretching of afferent arteriole causes reflex muscle contraction and reduces the diameter of arteriole and thus regulates the blood flow.

b. **Juxtaglomerular apparatus:** Juxtaglomerular apparatus is a group of cells located between the distal convoluted tubule and afferent arteriole. A fall in GFR activates juxtaglomerular cells to release renin and increase glomerular blood flow as well as GFR.

Selective Reabsorption

Most of the glomerular filtrates (99%) are selectively reabsorbed by capillary networks surrounding proximal convoluted tubules, loop of Henle and distal convoluted tubule. Selective absorption occurs by osmosis and active absorption.

Osmosis: Eight per cent water, 50% urea along with sodium and chloride are reabsorbed by osmosis.

Active absorption: Useful substances such as glucose and amino acids are returned back to blood by active absorption.

Active Tubular Secretion

Active tubular secretion takes place at distal convoluted tubule. Potassium, hydrogen ions, certain drugs and metabolic wastes such as ammonia and creatinine are actively secreted into the tubule.

DISEASES OF THE KIDNEY

Acute Renal Failure

Acute and sudden reduction in glomerular filtration rate is called acute renal failure. It is usually reversible.

Causes may be as follows:
- **Prerenal:** Due to severe and prolonged shock
- **Renal:** Due to damage of kidney
- **Postrenal:** Due to obstruction to the outflow of urine

Chronic Renal Failure

Chronic renal failure is also known as chronic kidney disease (CKD) and GFR is reduced to less than 20%. Selective reabsorption and tubular secretions are also grossly impaired. Kidney functions are grossly affected leading to the accumulation of waste materials, acidosis and electrolyte imbalance.

End-Stage Renal Failure

End-stage renal failure is not compatible with life, if patients are not treated with dialysis or renal transplants.

CHAPTER 11

Basic Physics Relevant to Operation Theatre Equipment

Physics is a natural science, used to describe the fundamental laws related to different equipment used in operation theatre.

According to modern physics, the matter is a substance that has inertia and occupies physical space. Matter consists of various types of particles with different mass and size. The three states of matter are solid, liquid and gas.

Solid: It is compact or dense material. Its molecules do not change their position hence, solid maintains its shape.

Liquid: Molecules are less dense and constantly moving and, therefore, it does not maintain the shape but takes the shape of the container.

Gas: Molecules are constantly moving and bumping on each other and on the walls of the container. Gas expands evenly and fills the entire space.

VAPOUR AND GASES

- Substance normally present in the gaseous state at room temperature and atmospheric pressure is called gas.
- Vapour is the gaseous substance which is normally available in liquid form at room temperature and pressure.

- **Vapour pressure:** From the surface of liquid, some molecules escape into atmosphere as vapour and exerts pressure on surface of the liquid and the wall of container. This is called vapour pressure.
- **Saturated vapour pressure:** Some of the molecules in vapour form re-enter into liquid. This process continues until the number of molecules enters and escapes from liquid reach at equilibrium. At this stage, vapour pressure is maximum for the temperature which is called **saturated vapour pressure.**

Boiling point: Saturated vapour pressure increases with temperature. The temperature at which saturated vapour pressure becomes equal to atmospheric pressure is called the boiling point. Vapour pressure depends upon the type of liquid and temperature. It is not affected by atmospheric pressure.

Boiling point is a temperature at which liquid is converted to vapour at any given pressure.

Freezing point: Temperature at which liquid is converted to solid at any given pressure is called freezing point.

Effects of pressure: Changes in pressure cause changes in boiling and freezing points of a substance.

Critical temperature: Increase of pressure or decrease in temperature produces liquefaction of gaseous substances. Critical temperature means the temperature above which gas cannot be liquefied by increasing pressure.

Critical pressure: Pressure required for liquefying gas at its critical temperature.

Flow of Gas through the Tube with Variable Diameters

When gas flows through a tube with gradually reducing diameter and finally leads to constriction, the velocity of gas should be highest at the point of constriction. According to Bernoulli principle, increase in velocity is associated with fall in pressure.

The Bernoulli principle: An increase in velocity of a gas is associated with the fall of its pressure.

The Venturi effect: Fall in velocity distal to constricted tube causes the increase in pressure.

Clinical Implications of Bernoulli Principle and Venturi Effect

Increased velocity of the gas at the site of constriction of tube causes fall in pressure may be up to sub-atmospheric level, due to Bernoulli effect. If the entrainment tube is added at the site of constriction, the air is sucked in through entrainment tube due to sub-atmospheric pressure (Fig. 11.1).

Nebulizer, Venturi masks and jet ventilator are based on these principles.

Gas Laws

Boyle's law: At a constant temperature, the volume of the fixed amount of gas varies inversely with its pressure.

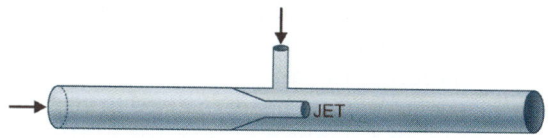

Fig. 11.1: Injector devices with entrainment port

$$PV = k \ or \ V \propto 1/P \ or \ P_1V_1 = P_2V_2 = P_3V_3$$

Charles' law: According to Charles' law at constant pressure, the volume of a gas is directly proportional to its absolute temperature.

$$V/T = k \ or \ V \propto T$$

Dalton's law: In a physical mixture of gases, each gas exerts same pressure which it exerts if occupied alone in the same volume of container. Pressure of the mixed gas equals the sum of partial pressure of the individual gases.

Thus in any mixture of gases, the partial pressure exerted by each gas is proportional to its fractional concentration.

$$P = P_1 + P_2 + P_3$$

Fick's law: Rate of diffusion of gases and liquids is proportional to the gradient of concentration. Whenever the differences in concentrations of a particular substance in a solution exist between the two sides of a semi-permeable layer, the diffusion occurs from higher to lower concentration.

Based on Fick's principles, cardiac output is measured. Total uptake or release of a substance by an organ is equal to the product of the blood flow to the organ and arterio-venous concentration difference of the substance.

$$\text{Cardiac output} = \frac{VO_2}{C_a - C_v}$$

Avogadro's law: Equal volume of all gases always contains an equal number of molecules under the same temperature and pressure.

One gram molecule of a gas occupies 22.4 litres at normal temperature and pressure. This is used to calculate the amount of volatile liquid needed to obtain a known percentage of vapour in a mixture of gases.

$$\frac{22.4 \times \text{Liquid density}}{\text{Molecular weight}} \times 1000 \ ml$$

BASIC SCIENCE RELATED TO DEFIBRILLATORS

Capacitors: Device that stores electrical charges is called a capacitor. It consists of two conducting plates separated by non-conducting materials.

Capacitance: The ability of the capacitor to store electrical charges is called capacitance.

Inductor: Inductor is an electrical component which opposes the current flow by the generation of an electromotive force.

Inductance measures the ability to generate resistance.

Charging of Defibrillator

During charging of defibrillator, switch is positioned to flow 5000 V DC. Current flows only in upper half of the circuit and thus charge is built upon the capacitor plates (Fig. 11.2).

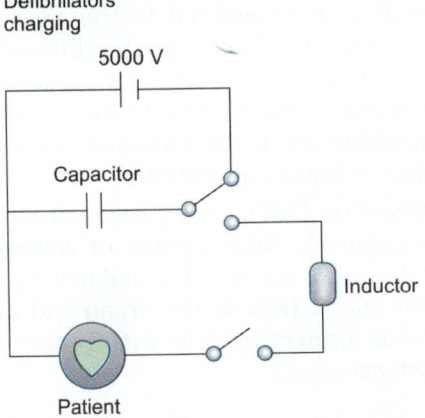

Fig. 11.2: Circuit during charging defibrillator

Discharging of Defibrillator

During discharging the defibrillator, upper as well as lower switches are closed. Stored current from capacitor is delivered to the patient. The inductor modifies the current to deliver (Fig. 11.3).

BASIC PRINCIPLES OF PULSE OXIMETRY

- Haemoglobin saturation of oxygen (SpO_2) is measured by differential absorption of red and infrared light in tissue.

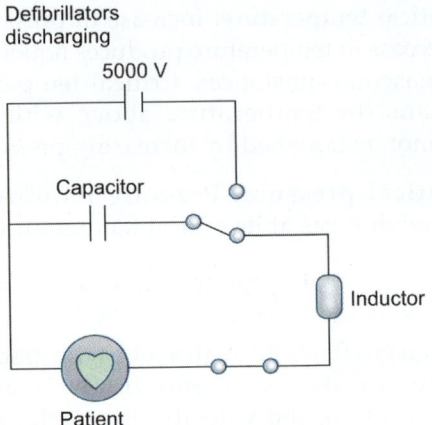

Fig. 11.3: Circuit during discharging defibrillator

- The red and infrared light delivered by the light source absorb, reduced and oxy-haemoglobin, respectively. Pulse oximeter assesses the ratio between absorption of these two rays and determines arterial oxygen saturation.

Basic Principles of Fiberoptic Endoscope

- Endoscope is used to examine the interior of the cavity through the small hole and perform necessary operative procedures.
- Based on the site of operation, it is called laparoscopy, arthroscopy, bronchoscopy or thoracoscopy.
- By these endoscopes, the surgeon visualizes the interior of the cavity and by cutting tools attached to such endoscope surgery is performed.
- Fiberoptic endoscope consists of bundles of optical fibers made up of plastic or glass. They carry information from the distal places using optical technology.

BASIC PRINCIPLES OF LASER

- Laser is a device that emits light through a process of optical amplification. LASER means "light amplification by stimulated emission of radiation".
- Laser is a narrow beam focused to very tiny spots and enabling laser for cutting or lithotripsy.

Section II

Operation Theatre

CHAPTER 12

Operation Theatre Planning and Management

Operation theatre or operation room is a specialized facility within a hospital where surgical procedures are done under a strict aseptic controlled environment.

Aim of Planning

- To promote high standards of asepsis
- To ensure the safety of patients and OT personnel
- To ensure optimum physical working conditions
- To ensure optimum utilization of operation theatre
- To facilitate co-ordinate services

PHYSICAL SET-UP

Location

- Operation theatre should be located at the place which is free from external disturbances and it should also allow the convenient and free flow of patients posted for operation.
- It should be close to the surgical ward, surgical intensive care unit and other supporting departments.

Number of Operation Theatre

Number of operation theatre depends upon the total number of surgical beds of a hospital.

Number of bed hospital	Number of OT for indoor patients		Number of OT for OPD and emergency patients	
	Minor	Major	Minor	Major
300	2	3	1	–
500	2	5	1	1
750	2	8	1	1
1000	2	10	1	1

Size of the Operation Theatre

- General operation room—40 sqm
- Specialized operation room—60 sqm (orthopedics, neurosurgery, cardiothoracic OT)
- Endoscopy procedure room and minor OT—20 sqm

ZONAL DISTRIBUTION OF OPERATION THEATRE

Operation theatre is divided into four zones to achieve the high degree of asepsis.

1. **Protective zone:** This is at the entrance of the operation theatre. Protective zone includes:
   - Patient reception and waiting area
   - Trolley bay
   - Changing room
   - Store room

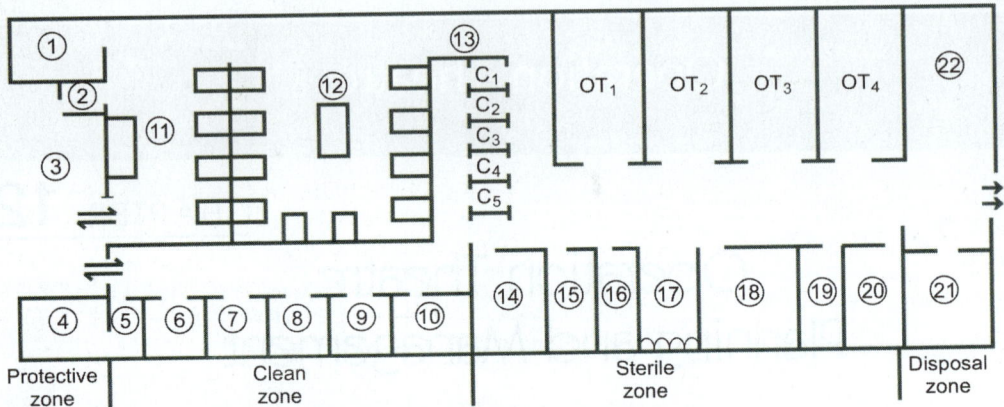

Protective zone: 2: Reception, 3: Patient waiting area, trolley bay, etc.

Clean zone : 1 and 4: Washroom, 5: Shoe changing room, 6: Pantry, 7: Room for administrator, 8: Doctors room, 9: Sister's room, 10: Store, 11: Preoperative room, 12: Recovery room, 13: Corridor for shifting of patient, C_1, C_2, C_3, and C_4: Changing room

Sterile zone: 14: Store, 15: OT administrator room, 16: Doctor room, 17: Scrup area, 18: Endoscopy room, 19: Trolley layout area, 20: Theatre sterilization unit. OT_1, OT_2, OT_3, and OT_4,: Operation theatre

Disposal zone: 21: Room for separation of different disposable item for disposal, 22: Room for cleaning of reusable item for sterilization

Fig. 12.1: Operation theatre layout

2. **Clean zone:** It connects the protective zone to the sterile zone. It includes:
   - Preoperative room
   - Recovery room
   - Storage for clean equipment
   - Service room for staff
   - Room for administrative staff
3. **Sterile zone:** Maintenance of the sterile environment is an essential aspect of this zone. It includes:
   - Operation room
   - Anaesthesia room
   - Scrubbing area
   - Instrument trolley layout area
4. **Disposal zone:** Disposal zone is used to dispose dirty linen, equipment and bio-medical waste. It includes:
   - Dirty room
   - Disposal corridor.

LAYOUT OF OPERATION THEATRE

Layout of operation theatre should be designed to establish four clear zones, where operation theatre staff should not pass through the unprotected or dirty zone (Fig. 12.1). It should facilitate to remove contaminated materials without passing through the clean or sterile zone.

DESIGN OF OPERATION ROOM

Doors
- Width should be at least 5 feet to facilitate easy transfer of trolley.
- Sliding doors are preferred.

Floor
- Strong and impermeable flooring with a minimum number of joints.
- It should be electroconductive to dissipate static electricity.

Walls
- The walls should be jointless, stainproof, waterproof, fireproof and non-reflective.
- It should be easy to wash and clean.

Light and Electricity

- Uninterrupted power supply with a generator and/or UPS back-up.
- Wall illuminated with florescent shadow less light.
- Recommended illuminations for the different zone of operation theatre:
  - Entire operation theatre: 400 lux
  - Operation room: 1,000 lux
  - Operative field: 50,000 lux

MODULAR OPERATION THEATRE

- It is a prefabricated structure made up of steel shell with a jointless sealed sterile coating. Sharp edges and corners are replaced by concave surface to prevent bacterial contamination and also to maintain better airflow. Flooring system is made antistatic.
- Modular OT is a modern concept of operation theatre, where all modern technology is introduced to provide the best possible care to all surgical patients. This includes modular ceiling light, pendants for different types of equipment, laminar flow, air purifier—HEPA filter and centralized cooling system. This ensures OT environment free from growth of pathogens.
- Advantages of modular operation theatre are:
  1. *Fast construction:* Construction of modular OT takes almost half time as compared to conventional technique because many parts of the building are delivered as a prefabricated structure.
  2. *Easy expansion and maintenance:* Modular OT can be expanded or modified very easily according to the need of the theatre.
  3. *Offer fire, noise, and radiation protection:* Walls, doors and windows are covered with lead shielding to ensure protection from radiation due to C-Arm and X-ray machine used in theatre.

Modular OT also takes complete protection against fire and noise.
  4. *Offer bacteria-free zone:* Antimicrobial agents are added on the surface during the manufacturing process and help to make the environment bacteria-free.

CLEANING, DECONTAMINATION AND STERILIZATION

Aim

- To clean operation theatre and remove contaminants, dust and organic matters.
- Disinfection of operation theatre and reduce the number of microbes.
- To reduce microbial count

Cleaning of Walls and Roof

- Do not disturb these areas unnecessarily.
- Frequent cleaning has very little effect.
- Clean only when good amount of dust is accumulated.
- Clean with vacuum cleaner to prevent aerosol spread.
- Thorough disinfection of operation theatre should be done after cleaning of walls and roof.

Cleaning and Disinfection of Floor

- Number of microbes on the floor depends upon the number and movement of persons within the theatre. However, only 1% of microbes are pathogenic or harmful for surgical patients.
- Do not use broom because it may cause aerosol spread. Clean the floor with vacuum cleaner only.
- Use of detergent reduces bacterial flora by 80% and addition of disinfectant reduces up to 95%.

Cleaning of Operation Theatre between the two Operative Procedures

- At the end of the surgical procedure, discard waste materials in the prescribed plastic bags. Biomedical waste should not be accumulated within theatre.

- Soiled gowns should not be discarded inside the theatre.
- In between the two operative procedures, operation table and other theatre equipment should be cleaned with the disinfectant solution.
- If there is spillage of blood or other body fluids, decontamination should be done with bleaching powder or chlorine water.

Cleaning of Operation Theatre at the End of the Day

- Clean all the tables, equipment, and door handles with detergent.
- Clean the floor with detergent. Use bleaching powder, if it is soiled with blood or other body fluids.
- Finally swab the floor with disinfectant like phenol in the concentration of 1:10.

STERILIZATION OF OPERATION THEATRE

Fumigation

- This is a traditional method of sterilization of operation theatre with a goal to achieve zero bacteria and spore environment.
- Formaldehyde vapour is generated when liquid formaldehyde is mixed with water and exposed to raised temperature (80°–90°C).
- Formaldehyde vapour decontaminates OT environment.

Method

- Switch off all the machines and electrical appliances.
- Close doors and windows and seal with adhesive tape.
- Measure the volume of operation theatre (L × B × H). Five hundred milliliter formaldehyde is required for 1000 cubic feet volume.
- Mix 500 ml formaldehyde with 1000 ml water in a fogging machine.
- Switch on the fogging machine in a closed theatre. Machine automatically stops after 45 minutes or a predetermined time.

- Seal the room for 24 hours.
- Neutralize residual formalin gas with ammonia.

MODERN APPROACH OF STERILIZATION

Modern technique has been developed with an intension to replace formaldehyde with non-toxic safe agents. Sterilization can be done much quicker than traditional method.

Bacillocid

- Formaldehyde-free disinfectant cleaner.
- Suitable for short-term disinfectant.
- Active ingredients are glutaral 100 mg/g, benzyl-C12-18-alkyldimethylammonium chloride 60 mg/g and didecyldimethylammonium chloride 60 mg/g.

Vikron

- It contains potassium peroxymonosulphate, sodium dodecylbenzene sulphonate, sulfamic acid and inorganic buffer.
- It is safe virucidal, bactericidal, fungicidal and microbactericidal.
- It can be used for sterilization of operation theatre.

Silver Nitrate and Hydrogen Peroxide

- It is 0.01% silver nitrate and 11% hydrogen peroxide.
- It does not have toxic effects like formaldehyde.
- It is virucidal, bactericidal, fungicidal and microbactericidal.
- It has a deep penetrating capacity.
- It is used with ultralow volume fogger machine that releases droplets of 7 to 20 μ.
- Droplets of germicidal solution trap the suspended particulate matters and kill the microorganism.
- Operation theatre can be sterilized in two hours.
- It can be done at the end of the day regularly.

CHAPTER 13

Surgical Microbiology and Antimicrobial Therapy

Microbiology is the branch of medical sciences that deals with the study of microorganisms such as bacteria, fungi, protozoa and viruses.

Microorganisms may be a natural resident of some organ systems such as the gastro-intestinal tract or respiratory tract of the human body. They are called resident florae.

When nonresident florae invade the susceptible organs of the human body, it is called infection. Sometimes resident florae may increase in huge numbers and produce pathological conditions.

Microorganisms causing infection are broadly classified into: Bacteria, viruses, fungi and protozoa.

BACTERIA

- Bacteria are unicellular structure; survive in different environments including the human body. There are more than 5,000 species of bacteria, which are classified according to their shape, life cycle and staining characteristics.
- They are microscopic structures of 0.5–5 µm length.
- They have DNA but no formal nucleus (prokaryotic) and no membrane-bound organelles.

Classification of Bacteria

- **According to shapes:**
  - *Bacilli:* Rod-shaped bacteria; such as *Escherichia coli.*
  - *Cocci:* Oval or spherical-shaped bacteria such as streptococci, staphylococci and pneumococci.
  - *Vibrios:* Comma-shaped bacteria, e.g. *Vibrio cholerae.*
  - *Spirochetes:* Spiral-shaped bacteria such as *Leptospira* and *Treponema pallidum*
  - *Actinomycetes:* Bacteria having branched filaments such as *Mycobacterium tuberculosis.*
  - *Pleomorphs:* Bacteria changes shape from rod to round and vice versa.

- **According to life cycle:**
  - *Aerobic:* Bacteria requiring oxygen for multiplications and survival is called aerobic bacteria.
  - *Anaerobic:* Anaerobic bacteria survive only in the absence of oxygen or when oxygen present in a very low concentration such as dead muscles.

- **According to staining characteristics:** There are two types of bacteria according to staining characteristics. Gentian violet solution is applied to the microorganism.

Cell wall of bacteria gets exposure to such a solution for sometimes and then washed with 95% alcohol and acetone. After this procedure, their staining character is analyzed.

- *Gram-positive bacteria:* Bacteria retain a dark-purple blue colour is called Gram-positive bacteria. Examples are *Streptococcus*, *Pneumococcus* and *Mycobacterium tuberculosis*.
- *Gram-negative bacteria:* Bacteria retain a stain of light pink after completions of Gram staining are called Gram-negative bacteria. Examples are *Escherichia coli*, *Neisseria meningitides*, *Salmonella*, *Shigella* and *Pseudomonas*.

VIRUS

- Viruses are microscopic structures smaller than bacteria. They are not independent cells, obligatory parasites. They live as intracellular parasites either in somatic cells of host or within bacteria.
- They are made up of either DNA or RNA but never both. DNA or RNA is covered by a membrane known as a capsid.
- They act by transfer of its DNA or RNA genome into the cell of host.
- Viruses of special interest for surgical patients are HIV, hepatitis B and hepatitis C.

FUNGI

- Fungi have a nucleus with a rigid cell wall. They are large branched organisms. According to morphology, fungi are classified into four groups:
  - Moulds
  - Yeasts
  - Yeast-like fungi
  - Dimorphic fungi
- Infection is transmitted by spores in direct contact with the respiratory system, mucous membrane or non-intact skin. Example,

Aspergillus fumigatus causes respiratory disease.

PROTOZOA

- Protozoa is a microscopic but relatively large size. They are single-cell microorganisms, without a morphologically distinct cell wall.
- Protozoans are transmitted by the ingestion of cyst through fecal-oral route.
- They are also transmitted by direct contact with organisms secreted by the mucous membrane of genitourinary tract.
- Amoebiasis by *Entamoeba histolytica* and hydratid cyst by *Echinococcus granulosus* are important from surgical point of view. Hydatid cyst is usually removed by surgery. Amoebiasis may cause intestinal perforation or liver abscess.

ANTIMICROBIAL THERAPY

Antimicrobial agents are chemical substances, act by inhibition of growth or cause death of microorganisms.

Antibiotic is the substance produced by microorganism or similar substances produced by chemical synthesis and cause the death of microorganisms.

Mechanism of Action

- Interfere with cell wall synthesis.
- Act on the cytoplasmic membrane and cause destruction of the cell membrane of microorganism.
- Inhibit protein synthesis.
- Inhibit DNA function.
- Acts as a metabolic antagonist.

Antibiotics act either by killing bacteria (bactericidal) or inhibiting the growth of bacteria (bacteriostatic). Antibiotics do not attack other cells of body because they do not recognize higher-order cell walls and advanced synthesis of human cells. For this reason, cells of the human body remain unaffected by antibiotics.

According to the mechanism of actions of antibiotics, they are classified in the following groups (Tables 13.1 to 13.3).

Table 13.1	Antibiotics inhibit cell wall synthesis of bacteria and produce bactericidal effect			
S. no.	Category and names of antibiotics	Type of bacteria	Side effects	Remarks
1.	Penicillins group Amoxicillin Ampicillin Augmentin Carbenicillin	Gram-positive	Hypersensitivity reaction Haemolytic anaemia Interstitial nephritis	Narrow spectrum Safe in pregnancy
2.	Cephalosporin group 1st Cephalexin 2nd Cefuroxime 3rd Rocephin 4th Cefepime	Gram-positive Gram-negative	Colitis	Broad-spectrum Used in surgical prophylaxis Safe in pregnancy
3.	Carbapenems Doripenem Ertapenem Imipenum	Gram-positive Gram-negative	Excreted through kidney	Broad-spectrum Good for anaerobes
4.	Glycopeptides Vancomycin	Gram-positive	Ototoxic Nephrotoxic	Narrow spectrum
5.	Polypeptides Bacitracin Polymyxin Colistin Neomycin	Gram-positive Gram-negative	–	Topical prophylaxis for skin infection

Table 13.2	Antibiotics act by inhibition of protein synthesis			
S. no.	Category and names of antibiotics	Action	Side effects	Remarks
1.	Macrolides Erythromycin Azithromycin Clidamycin	Bacteriostatic	Jaundice Hepatitis Cardiac QT prolong	Broad-spectrum Used in lung infection
2.	Tetracyclines Doxycycline Minocycline	Bacteriostatic	Discolour teeth and bones Nephrotoxicity Not used in pregnancy	Broad-spectrum

Contd.

Table 13.2	Antibiotics act by inhibition of protein synthesis (Contd.)			
S. no.	Category and names of antibiotics	Action	Side effects	Remarks
3.	**Aminoglycosides** Gentamicin Tobramycin Neomycin Kanamycin	Bactericidal	Nephrotoxic Ototoxic Aggravate myasthenia gravis	Broad-spectrum Used for treating septicemia Meningitis
4.	**Lincosamide** Clindamycin	Bacteriostatic	Decrease effectiveness of oestrogen con-traceptives	Broad-spectrum for anerobes Treats protozoa, toxoplasmosis, osteomyelitis, intra-abdominal sepsis

Table 13.3	Antibiotics inhibit nucleic acid synthesis and replication of bacteria and produce bactericidal effects			
S. no.	Category and names of antibiotics	Type of bacteria Gram +/−	Side effects	Remarks
1.	**Ansamycin** Rifampin	+/−	Hepatotoxic Skin pigmentation	Indicated in TB, leprosy and osteomyelitis
2.	**Fluoroquinolones** Cinoxacin Ciprofloxacin Levofloxacin	+	Phototoxicity Drug interaction with theophylline, anticonvulsant drugs	Renal excretion
3.	**Sulphonamides** Bactrim (bacteriostatic)	+	Blood dyscrasia	Used in urinary tract infection
4.	**Nitroimidazole** Metronidazole	+/−	Peripheral neuropathy Intolerance to alcohol	Good for anaerobes; trichomoniasis, giardia
5.	Isoniazid	Micobacterial inhibitor	–	Used in tuberculosis

The incidence of hypersensitivity reactions is high. Therefore, before of the administration of antibiotics, patients should be enquired about the history of any drug allergy. They should be the closely monitored for any evidence of allergy after the administration of drugs.

Antibiotics in the Perioperative Period

Use of antibiotics has reduces the incidence of postoperative infection and made the surgical procedure safer. However, perioperative antibiotic therapy is adjuvant not the substitutes of aseptic or sterile techniques.

Guidelines of Perioperative Antibiotics Therapy

- In grossly contaminated or infected surgical cases, the choice of antibiotics and duration of therapy depend upon the type of pathogen (culture and sensitivity test), severity as well as the site of infection and clinical response of therapy.

- **Antibiotic prophylaxis:** Prophylactic use of antibiotics attack microorganism before colonization takes place at the target tissue. Prophylactic antibiotics are administered 30 minutes to one hour before surgical incision and it is continued for 24 hours.

- **Prophylactic antibiotics are commonly used in the following scenario:**
  - Erythromycin ophthalmic ointment 0.5% for neonatal ophthalmic prophylaxis immediately after birth by normal delivery or the caesarean section.
  - Procedures associated with brief exposure to possible infection (cystitis after cystoscopy).
  - Procedures associated with the high risk of infection such as surgery for biliary tract obstruction or transection of the colon.
  - Procedures are commonly not associated with infection but infections, if occur, cause life-threatening consequences. Total joint replacement, cardiac valve replacement or vascular graft.
  - Intraoperative irrigation of surgical site with antibiotics to minimize bacterial colonization. Intraperitoneal or intrapleural instillation of antibiotics such as bacitracin diluted in normal saline or Ringer lactate.

Selection of Antibiotics

It depends upon:

- Site of surgical procedure
- Potential pathogens found at the site
- Patient history of drug allergy, if any
- Patients co-morbid conditions especially deranged renal or liver function

Procedure of Antibiotic Prophylaxis

- Parenteral antibiotic prophylaxis should be started 1–2 hours prior to surgery.
- In most of the surgical cases, it is desirable to limit the duration of administration of antibiotics within 12 hours.
- The use of parenteral antibiotics increases the risk of antibiotic toxicity. Therefore, it should not be continued beyond 48 hours.
- In cases of caesarean section, a prophylactic antibiotic is administered after clamping of the placental cord.
- Oral prophylactic antibiotic is sometimes used before colorectal surgery. They should be stopped 24 hours before surgery and switched over to parenteral preparation.
- There is no role of prophylactic oral antibiotics as continuation or supplementation of parenteral antibiotics in the postoperative period.
- Topical antibiotics should not cause any serious local or systemic side effects.

CHAPTER 14

Principles of Sterile Technique

Term 'sterile' means free from living micro-organism including spore. It is different from the terminology 'asepsis' which means absence of microorganism that causes disease.

Sterile field: It is the area around surgical incision over the draped patient on the table. This area includes operative field, furniture covered with sterile drapes and all personnel who are properly attired in sterile garb.

Sterile technique: Technique by which contamination with microorganism is prevented. Sterile technique includes many processes associated with asepsis but at a higher degree.

APPLICATIONS OF STERILE TECHNIQUE

Sterile technique is applied under the following conditions.

- Preparation of an invasive procedure by sterilization of necessary instruments and materials.
- Preparation of the sterile team by scrubbing, gowning and gloving.
- Preparation and maintenance of the sterile field by preparation of skin and draping by sterile materials.
- Maintenance of sterility throughout the surgical procedures.

BASIC PRINCIPLES

- **Only sterile items are used in the sterile field:** Sterile instruments, draping materials, surgical mops and sponges used in the operative field must be obtained from sterile zone. If there is any doubt about sterility, materials should not be used for the operation. There is a saying, "When in doubt throw it out".
  - Consider unsterile:
    - If the sterilized package is found in a non-sterile zone.
    - If an unsterile person comes in close contact with a sterile table.
    - If the integrity of package material is not intact.
    - If the sterile package wrapped in a material other than plastics or moisture resistant materials and becomes wet.
    - If the sterile package wrapped in a piece of muslin and drops to the floor.
- **Parts of gown considered sterile:**
  - In front from chest to level of sterile field and sleeves from above elbows to cuffs.
  - Hands should be kept above the level of the waist or on the sterile field.

- Hands should be kept away from mouth and body.
- Elbows are kept close to side.

• **Only top of tables are sterile:**
- Only the top of the table draped with draping materials is sterile. Sides of drapes extending below the table are considered unsterile.
- Anything falls at the edge of the table is unsterile.
- During the unfolding of sterile drape, the part that drops below the table surface is considered unsterile and it should not be brought back to the table.

• **Sterile team touch only sterile items:**
- Scrub assistance should maintain contact with the sterile field only.
- Circulating assistants should not directly contact the sterile field.
- Sterile items wrapped in the packet are brought by a circulating nurse and open wrappers on sterile zone.

• **Unsterile person should avoid to reach over a sterile field:**
- Unsterile circulating assistant should never reach over a sterile field to transfer sterile items
- Circulating assistants should stand at a distance from the sterile zone specially during:
  ▪ Delivery of sterile items
  ▪ Adjusting the operation theatre light
  ▪ Operating the C-arm
- Scrub operating team must drape a non-sterile table towards self first to protect them from the unsterile zone.

• **Edges of any packet that encloses the sterile contents are considered unsterile:**
- Many sterile items used during operation are available in package. During operation, package is opened by circulating assistance and supply the materials present within that package. During opening of

packages, a margin of safety should be maintained. The insides of wrappers are considered sterile up to within 1 inch of edges.
- Edges of the package are unsterile up to 1 inch from the margins.
- Sterile person lifts contents from packages.
- Package should be pulled back and contents should be lifted upwards or flipped.
- When sterile bottle is opened, content must be used or discarded

• **Time of creating sterile field:**
- Sterile field for operation should be created just before the operation. Delay increases the chances of infections.
- Covering a sterile table for later use is not recommended.

• **Observation of sterile area:**
- When the sterile field is set up, it should be constantly monitored to maintain sterility.
- Unmonitored fields may become unsterile by unintentional touch or interference.

• **Sterile persons are safe in sterile zone:**
- Sterile persons should stand at a safe distance from the operating table during draping the patient.
- Sterile persons should turn back to non-sterile person or areas while crossing that area.
- Sterile persons should cross each other by attaining back-to-back position.
- Sterile person should face the sterile area during any movement.
- Movement around the sterile area should be minimum to avoid contamination of sterile area.

• **Minimum contact to sterile area by sterile persons:**
- Sterile persons should not lean on sterile tables or draped patient.
- Sitting or leaning of the sterile person against a non-sterile area is not allowed.

- **Maintain a distance from the sterile area by an unsterile person:**
  - Unsterile persons must maintain a distance of at least 30 cm from sterile area.
  - Unsterile person should not pass between the two sterile zones.
  - Movements of circulating assistance should be restricted to minimum near the sterile area.
- **Preservation of integrity of sterile packages:**
  - Sterile packages should be laid on dry surfaces to prevent contamination.
  - If sterile package becomes wet, it should be discarded.
  - Draping materials should be placed on the dry fields.
  - If draping material gets wet, it should be covered by impermeable sterile materials.
  - Sterile packages should be stored in the dry clean area.
  - Sterile packages should be handled with sterile dry hand or forceps.
- **Maintain the number of microorganism to minimum irreducible level, where complete sterilization is not possible.**
  - Sterilization of skin is not possible, so use the antiseptic measures to minimize the number of microorganisms.
  - Scrubbing of certain areas is not possible such as mouth, nose, throat or anus. Number of microorganisms is high in these areas. So attempt to clean periphery first and then areas with high numbers of microorganism. Sponge once used for cleaning the area with high micro-organism should be discarded immediately.
  - If the operative area is grossly infected as in case of debridement or amputation, steps must be taken to prevent the spread of infection due to contamination.

CHAPTER 15

Operation Theatre Attire,
Surgical Scrub, Gowning and Gloving

Main object of the operation room procedure is to perform safe surgery without any infection of the operative wound. Therefore, all persons entering in theatre complex should be in theatre clothes (not street clothes) and must wear cap, mask and OT shoes. Those who are involved in the surgical procedures must follow the standard technique of scrubbing, gowning and gloving. This art is very important to prevent postoperative infection.

THEATRE ATTIRE

- This is a professional dress used by the persons (like doctors, nurses, technicians, cleaners) entering the OT complex.
- It has one short-sleeved shirt and one pant. This dress is clean and replaces the street clothes which is more contaminated.
- Enough attire is kept in the changing rooms in different sizes. Some hospitals have different dress colour for different categories of staff for easy identification.
- It is washed and laundered after each use (Fig. 15.1).

FACE MASK

Face mask prevents the free passage of organisms from nose and mouth to the exterior and vice versa. Usually, it is available in sterile pack. It has four strings.

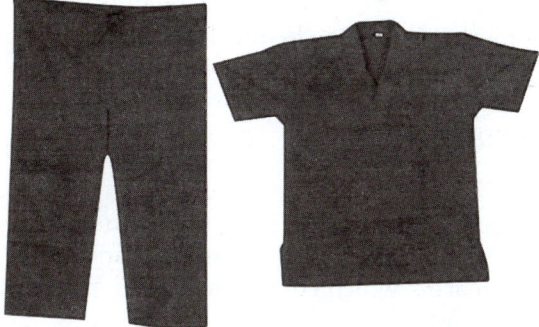

Fig. 15.1: Operation theatre dress

Method of Wearing the Mask

- Choose a sterile mask only to use.
- The upper two strings should be tied behind the head and above the ears.
- Lower two strings must be tied in a similar way but below the ears.
- Ensure that it has covered your mouth and nose properly and the expired air is filtered through the mask. Idea is that the organisms coming from the respiratory tract will not be able to come to the air in front.
- Do not keep it for more than 3–4 hours at a stretch. Otherwise, concentration of organisms in the mask will be increased after long hours of use (Fig. 15.2).

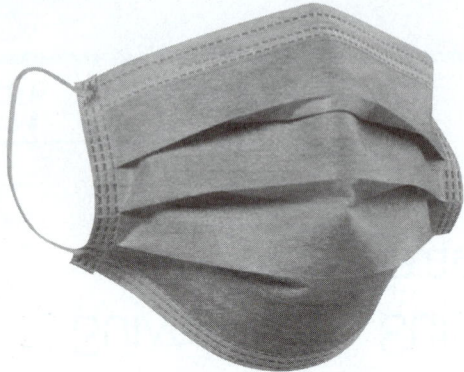

Fig 15.2: Front and side view of face mask

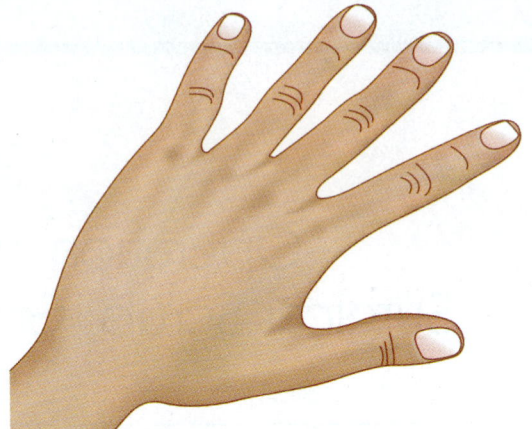

Fig 15.3: Areas of hands with high concentration of organisms

SURGICAL SCRUBBING

Scrubbing is one of the most important measures to prevent surgical site infection. It is mechanical and chemical washing of the hands of persons by which the dirt and microorganisms present in the skin is reduced in large numbers.

Objects of Scrubbing

- Removal of dirt, sweat and skin scales containing bacteria from the hands and forearms which contaminates the surgical wound.
- The microorganism present in the hands especially in the nail folds and web spaces is not transferred to the operative wound.

Key Points for Effective Scrubbing

- Running tap water in wash basin with a long handle stopper
- Soap
- Chlorhexidine/povidone-iodine liquid
- Soft nail brush (preferred sterile)
- Sterile towel
- Hand disinfectant (Fig. 15.3)

Method

- Check the nails, it should be short.
- Check any cut, abrasion, burn or any infective lesion in hands and forearm. That might contaminate the operative wound more.

- Remove jewellery and nail polish.
- Apply soap over hands, forearms up to the area just above the elbow. Then wash under running tap water after a few seconds.
- Repeat the above procedure 3 to 5 times and brush the digital web space and nail folds where normal washing cannot remove the organisms easily.
- Chlorhexidine/povidone-iodine is also used for chemical washing. Repeated application of chemicals and soap followed by washing is recommended (Fig. 15.4).
- Use sterile towel to remove extra water from the hands and forearms, but do not touch the unwashed areas of the body or any other object with hands at this stage. It is better to take two sterile towels for drying two hands.
- To make scrubbing more effective, use hand disinfectant over washed areas and keep it for 45 seconds to 1 minute to kill and reduce the number of organisms.
- Whole washing procedure should take at least 5 to 7 minutes, or more depending on contamination of hands and type of surgery.
- Hands should remain elevated and kept away from the body and mouth after washing till proceeds for gowning.

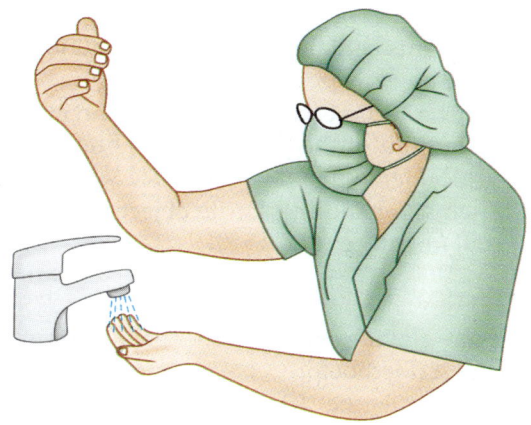

Fig 15.4: Hand wash

GOWNING

- Gown covers the body and limbs of the scrubbed surgical team member. The organisms from skin surface usually cannot pass through small pores of gown to contaminate the operative field.
- Ideally, the gown material should be impermeable to reduce chance of contamination.
- Gowns before sterilization are folded in such a way that the inner surface remains open and while unfolding the neck part with strings can be identified easily.
- After scrubbing only, the surgical team should proceed for wearing sterile gown.
- The sterile gown is necessary for any surgical procedure where the living tissue remains open and the surgical team members touch that area or its surroundings.

Objects of Wearing the Sterile Gown

- During operative procedure, any part of the body of surgeon or assistant may touch the operative area and there is a chance of contamination. To prevent such contamination, the use of a sterile gown is necessary.
- Normally our body secretes sweat which contains bacteria coming from the sweat gland. The sweat can percolate through the garment, but sterile impermeable gown does not allow sweat to contaminate the surgical field.
- Surgical team members with sterile gown have enough freedom to move around the operative field.
- Back flap of the gown can provide extra protection towards touching the instrument trolley inadvertently (Fig. 15.5).

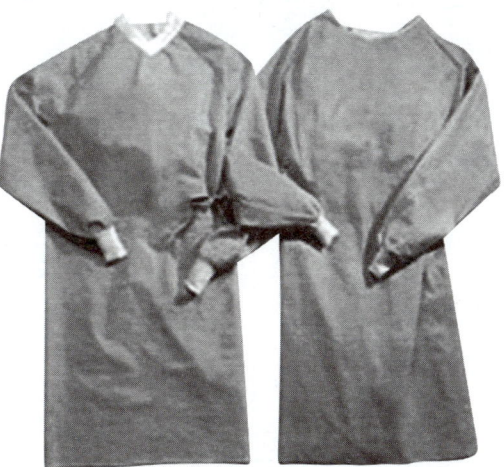

Fig 15.5: Showing back flap of the gown

Technique of Gowning

- Before gowning put the sterile hand gloves recommended by many authors.
- Grasp and unfold the gown with gloved hands (ensures less chance of contamination).
- Hold the gown with two hands at the level of the head but away from mouth and body.
- Try to find out the arm holes. Negotiate hands through arm holes and extend the forearm and elbow slowly with a gentle shake. The circulating nurse will help at this stage by pulling the neck and back strings of the gown and tie other back strings from behind.
- Tighten the wrist strings one by one.
- Put another pair of sterile hand gloves covering the wrist strings.

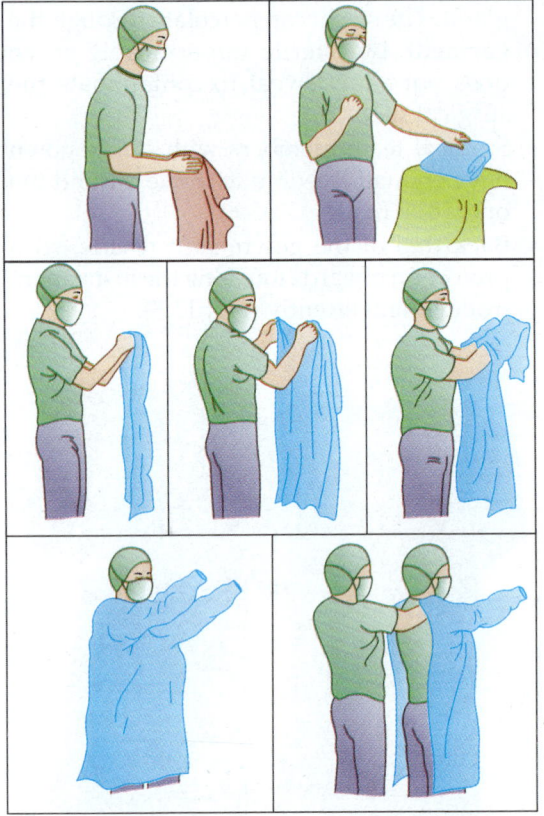

Fig 15.6: Technique of gowning

- Loosen the knot of back flap usually kept on the left side of the gown. The circulating nurse will hold it with sterile forceps and then make a half turn to your right side and tighten the strings around your waist. Now back is covered with a sterile flap (Fig. 15.6).

STERILE GLOVING

Sterile gloves in hands act as a barrier between the hand and the operative field. Gloves come in direct contact with the surgical wounds. They are available in sterile condition in a sterile double pack with a mark left and right. The cuff of the gloves is folded in a way that the inner surface remains exposed. Faulty technique of gloving causes loss of its sterility.

Objects

- It prevents contamination of the wound by the organisms present in the fingers.
- It prevents direct contact of blood and other tissue fluid of the patient to the fingers of surgical team members and vice versa.
- It helps in handling sterile objects without contaminating (Fig. 15.7).

Technique of Gloving

- Before gloving, ensure proper hand washing as described before.
- Hands must be dried properly and if not shake it in the air for a few seconds.
- The circulating nurse will open the package by separating and peeling apart the sides. The inner pack containing gloves is now pulled out and kept on a sterile platform.
- Grasp the cuff of the glove touching the folded part only by one hand and put your opposite thumb and other fingers to the proper space of the glove.
- Now insert four fingers of the gloved hand into the folded cuff of the other hand so as to touch its outer surface only.

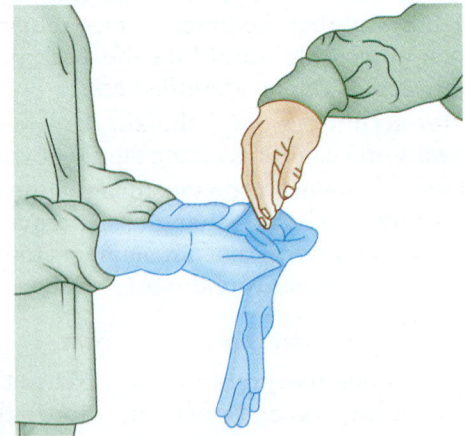

Fig 15.7: Technique of gloving. One hand holding the inner surface of the glove and the other hand is being negotiated without touching the outer sterile surface of the glove

- Insert your fingers of other hand into the respective spaces of the fingers and thumb.
- Unfold the cuff of the gloves touching its outer surface only and cover wrist strings.
- If fingers are not fitted in the proper space, it can be adjusted by pulling the gloves upwards.
- Care should be taken not to touch any part of the outer surface of the gloves during this procedure.
- One should practice the technique of gloving with unsterile gloves many times to make it easy.
- Gloves after use should be thrown in the bin marked for rubber goods.

PREPARATION OF INSTRUMENT TROLLEY

The top of the instrument trolley is not sterile, but sterile materials including instruments and linen required for operations need to be kept on the trolley. Top of the trolley is prepared aseptically to use as a sterile platform during surgery.

Objects

- To create a sterile work station where the scrubbed person can keep sterile items and handle instruments and other things aseptically and comfortably.
- Surgeon and assistants can keep sterile materials safely so that the items will not fall on the ground easily as the trolley has a low height guard railing.
- No need of asking circulating nurse repeatedly to bring supplies from the sterile store for that operation.

Method

- Before washing hands, swab the trolley top with antiseptic lotion and make it dry.
- Wash your hands. Put on sterile gloves and gown by standard technique. Use of back flap is important to remember otherwise unsterile and uncovered back may touch the sterile objects of the trolley.
- Put a sterile rubber sheet or any sterile impermeable cloth on the top and sides of the trolley. This is called the foundation layer.
- Circulating nurse opens the sterile drum containing sterile sheets of different sizes and can deliver the sheets as per requirement in that operation.
- Take one long sheet to cover the trolley top and all sides and the edge of the linen will extend up to the level little above the floor.
- Unfolding and spreading of the sheet should be done in a way that there remains no chance of touching any unsterile part of the trolley or any object of the surroundings.
- Now transfer the rest of the linen and instruments directly from the sterile drum to the trolley. The circulating nurse can also do it with transfer forceps.
- Heavy and big size items are sterilized separately using double or triple-layered clothe. This type of sterile pack is first placed over another trolley by the nurse who will open the first layer aseptically and the rest of the layers will be opened by the scrubbed person. Carefully transfer the actual sterile item without its wrapping to the sterile trolley.
- Remember some instruments and surgical items are common to all operations. So common items are displayed first as follows:
  - At least three empty pots, one kidney tray, three sponge-holding forceps and the bunch of gauze pieces are kept at one end of the table.
  - Two or three scalpels blade with handle of different sizes are kept in a separate small tray.
  - Sterile draping sheets of different sizes are placed at another end.
  - Bunch of artery forceps, tissue forceps, towel clip along with toothed and non-toothed thumb forceps, needle holder, pair of scissors are kept in the table for easy identification and use.

- The prepared instrument trolley may be covered with another sterile draping sheet if it is not used immediately. It can be opened later in a way that any unsterile part of the sheet does not touch the trolley top while lifting.

Special Precaution

- While preparing the instrument trolley try to avoid touching or holding its periphery which is always considered as less sterile because the non-scrubbed persons in the theatre might have touched the edges of the table inadvertently.
- The center of the table should be considered as the most sterile area for the same reason.
- Do not stand with hands supporting on the trolley.
- Your uncovered back should not touch the trolley

CHAPTER 16

Sterilization of Instruments and CSSD

Pathogenic microorganisms normally do not invade healthy tissue. However, it may cause infection, if mechanically introduced into the body. Therefore, instruments used for operative procedures are made absolutely microorganism free either by sterilization or disinfection.

STERILIZATION

Sterilization is the process by which all pathogenic and non-pathogenic microorganisms and endospores are killed. Sterilizers are the equipment used for sterilization of surgical instruments either by physical or chemical process.

Disinfection

Disinfection is the chemical or physical process that destroys most of the pathogenic microorganisms except bacterial endospores. The degree of disinfection depends on the strength of the agent and type of decontamination.

Antiseptics

Agents that prevent infection by destruction or inhibition of pathogens are called antiseptics.

Steps of Sterilization

- Decontamination includes cleaning all reusable items and disposing of disposable items as per the guidelines of biomedical waste management.
- Packaging and labelling of items kept for sterilization
- Loading and unloading of sterilizer
- Sterilization of items as per predetermined technique and duration
- Adhering to safety precautions
- Transport of sterile package to the sterile storage room
- Storing sterile items
- Transfer of sterile items from the storage area to a sterile field at the point of use under full aseptic precautions

METHODS OF STERILIZATION

Sterilization is either a physical or chemical process. Each has its advantages and disadvantages. Different methods used for sterilization of surgical instruments can be broadly classified under the following heading.

- Thermal (physical):
  - Steam under pressure
  - Dry heat

- Chemical:
  - Ethylene oxide gas
  - Formaldehyde gas
  - Hydrogen peroxide vapour
  - Ozone gas
  - Glutaraldehyde solution
  - Hypochlorus acid
- Radiation (physical):
  - Microwave sterilization
  - Gamma-ray and beta particle sterilization

Thermal Sterilization

Pasteurization

- Instruments are immersed at a high temperature for a specific time. Contact time is inversely related to temperature. Higher the temperature, lesser is the contact time.
- Commonly instruments are kept for 30 minutes at 70°C.
- Pasteurization has been used for sterilizations of the breathing system, reservoir bags, stylet, laryngoscope blades, etc.
- Advantages: Lower temperature is less damaging to equipment.

Autoclave

- This is a method of sterilization where the surgical items are exposed to heat above 100°C under pressure to make them germ-free.
- The boiling point of water is increased under pressure. This principle is used in an autoclave.
- Moist heat causes destruction of microorganisms by denaturation of macromolecules, primarily proteins. Destruction of cells by lysis may also play a role. While 'sterility' implies the destruction of free-living organisms that may grow within a sample, sterilization does not necessarily entail the destruction of infectious matter.

- Steam above 100°C is a better sterilization agent than dry heat or boiling at 100°C. Steam when condenses to water releases the latent heat, which is responsible for killing the bacteria. Sterilization by steam under pressure is carried out at temperature of 108°C to 147°C.
- Use of the autoclave is to sterilize culture media, rubber material, gown, dressings.
- **Mechanism of an autoclave:** The cylinder of the autoclave is filled with the sufficient amount of water. The objects are kept on the tray above the water with sufficient space between them. The electrically operated heater is then switched on. Safety valve is adjusted to ensure the desired pressure.
- Once the water starts to boil, the air–steam mixture is allowed to escape, as the temperature of this mixture is lower than the temperature of the steam. Once the air inside the cylinder is completely displaced by the steam, the discharge tap is closed. As the steam pressure increases, the excess steam escapes through the safety valve. Holding time of the autoclave (15 minutes at 121°C/ 10 minutes at 126°C/ 3 minutes at 134°C) is to be calculated from this point onwards.
- The autoclave is allowed to cool slowly till the pressure reaches the atmospheric pressure and the discharge tap is opened to allow entry of air.
- It must be kept in mind, not to open the tap when the internal pressure is high. This will lead to sudden boiling of the water and may even explode. Similarly, if it is opened when the pressure has gone below the atmospheric pressure, then an excessive amount of water will evaporate.
- Sterilization control is indicated by the appearance of green colour in a Browne's tube, when exposed at 121°C for 15 minutes in the autoclave.

Dry Heat Sterilization

- Destroys or kills microorganisms by protein denaturation, by oxidizing molecules, destroying cell components and increasing the levels of electrolytes.
- Dry heat is mostly used for sterilizing metal equipment, operative instruments.
- Use of direct flame of the Bunsen burner to sterilize forceps, inoculating loops is the easiest and most readily available method of sterilization.
- Incineration is a form of destruction of materials especially waste material, by burning. It is mostly used for treating biomedical wastes.
- The most widely used method of sterilization by dry heat is the use of a hot-air oven.
  - Here sterilization is achieved by conduction in an electrically heated chamber. Even the distribution of the heat inside the chamber is maintained by a fan.
  - 160°C for 2 hours or 170°C for 1 hour or 180°C for 30 minutes are the various holding times used for sterilization.
  - Articles and instruments inside the chamber should be arranged in a manner to allow free flow of the a hot air.
  - Heat is absorbed by the surface of the material initially and then heats the core of the material to reach the desired temperature.
  - Oven must be allowed to cool down over a period of 2 hours before opening. This is done to allow the glasswares to cool off slowly and prevents them from cracking due to sudden or uneven cooling.

Radiation Sterilization

Two types of radiation are used in sterilization: Non-ionizing—low energy infrared and ultraviolet rays; and ionizing—high energy gamma rays, X-rays and the high energy electrons.

Non-Ionizing Radiation

- These act by denaturation of the bacterial protein and interference with DNA replication. Infrared is mostly used for mass sterilization of syringes and catheters.
- Ultraiolet rays with a wavelength of 240 – 280 nm are bactericidal. UV rays are used to disinfect enclosed areas such as the bacteriological laboratory, inoculation hoods, laminar flows and operation theaters.

Ionizing Radiation

- These are highly penetrating in nature. Damages the bacterial DNA. As there is no appreciable rise of temperature with these rays, hence also referred as 'cold sterilization'.
- Due to the very high penetration ability, can sterilize materials through the outer packages and wrappings.
- Used to sterilize disposable items like plastic syringes, swabs, cannulas, catheters, culture plates.

Chemical Sterilization

A number of chemicals are used for sterilization or as disinfectants.

- The characteristics of an ideal disinfectant are:
  - It should not cause local or systemic toxicity.
  - Must not be a local irritant.
  - It should be cheap and easily available. Must be easy to use in all situations.
  - A wide spectrum of activity, including activity against bacteria, viruses, protozoa and fungi.
  - Activity in the presence of organic matters.
  - It should be quick-acting with high penetration power.
  - It must be stable and effective in both acidic and alkaline conditions.
  - Should not be corrosive to metals.

- Ethylene oxide is effective against all microorganisms including viruses and spores. It alters DNA and RNA structures. Because of its highly penetrating nature, it is used to sterilize plastic syringes and prepackaged materials. It is also used to sterilize plastic and rubber materials, heart – lung machines, sutures, etc.
- Hydrogen peroxide acts by releasing hydroxyl radicals. At 10–25% concentration, it has cidal activity against all microbes including spores. It is used to sterilize contact lenses, surgical prostheses and plastic implants.
- Ethyl alcohol and isopropyl alcohol are the most widely used variants of alcohol. Mostly used as a bactericidal (denaturing bacterial proteins). They have activity against tubercle bacilli but are not active against spores and viruses. Used as 60–70% concentration for skin asepsis.
- Commonly used antiseptics are derivatives of phenol, like cresols (lysol), chlorhexidine (savlon is a mixture of chlorhexidine and cetrimide), chloroxylenol. Cresols are used for sterilizing infected glasswares, scrubbing and cleaning of floors, disinfection of excreta. Chlorhexidine, in form of savlon is used for cleaning wounds, preoperative disinfection of the skin, bladder irritant (Table 16.1).

CENTRAL STERILE AND SUPPLY DEPARTMENT (CSSD)

Sterilization department is a very crucial department of a hospital. It is responsible for receiving, storing, processing, distributing and controlling the supplies of sterile equipment for the entire hospital under strict quality control.

Objectives

- To supply sterilized items to the entire hospital.
- To maintain and improve infection control measures.

Table 16.1	Common sterilization procedure for commonly used materials
Material	**Method**
Glasswares including glass syringes, histo-pathological containers	Hot-air oven
Disposable syringes and other disposable items	Gamma radiation
Cystoscope, laparoscope and endoscope Rubber, plastic and polythene tubings	Glutaraldehyde
Soiled dressings	Incineration
Skin	Alcohol, Savlon, povidone iodine
Aprons, dressings, metallic surgical instruments except sharp instruments	Autoclave
Sharp instruments	5% cresol (phenol derivative)
Operation theatre	Formaldehyde gas

- To reduce nosocomial infection in hospital
- To provide training of the sterilization process to nursing and paramedical personnel.

Location

It should be located near casualty ward, operation theatre, labour room and critical care unit. CSSD should have an adequate supply of water, steam, compressed air and uninterrupted electricity.

Size of CSSD

Number of bed of hospital	Size of CSSD
>250 beds	7 sq ft/bed
150–249 beds	8 sq ft/bed
100–149 beds	9 sq ft/bed
Below 100 beds	10 sq ft/bed

Layout: Basic Principle

- No back tracking of sterile goods. Separate receiving and issue counter.
- The receiving counter must be away from the issue counter.
- One way movement from receiving counter to issue counter.

Basic Divisions of CSSD

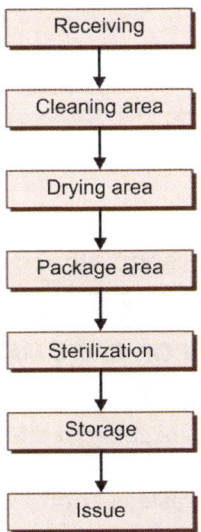

Equipment of CSSD

- Cleaning area
  - Washer disinfector
  - Hot-air ovens for drying instruments
  - Wall fixtures for drying
- Sterilization area
  - Steam sterilizer
  - Autoclave
  - Ethylene oxide
- Storage and distribution
  - Cub boards
  - Selves and racks
  - Trolleys and instruments tray

Staff Pattern

- CSSD supervisor
- CSSD attendant
- CSSD technician
- Boiler attendant
- Clerk
- Safaiwala

Central sterile and supply department plays a crucial role in any hospital. It takes a major role in the implementation of infection control policy in all departments and thus improves patient's safety.

CHAPTER 17

Biomedical Waste Management

BIOMEDICAL WASTE

Medical care is essential to life but it generates an enormous amount of waste which poses serious health hazards, if not properly disposed. Indiscriminate disposal results in a direct threat to the health of patients, the medical personnel and the environment. To avoid these health hazards, each waste requires specific treatment and management before final disposal.

Definition

According to **Biomedical Waste (Management and Handling) Rules, 1998** of India, "any **waste** which is generated during the diagnosis, treatment or immunization of human beings or animals or in research activities pertaining thereto or in the production or testing of biological".

The biomedical waste management rules 2018 are applicable to all persons who generate, collect, receive, store, transport, treat, dispose or handle the biomedical waste materials.

Occupier

Administrator of the institution (hospital, nursing home, clinics, etc.) generating the biomedical waste is called occupier.

Operator

Person owns or controls the biomedical waste treatment facility is called the operator.

CLASSIFICATION OF WASTE MATERIALS

According to WHO:
- 85% of all waste generated by hospitals is a general waste.
- Biomedical waste is approximately 10%.
- 5% is other type of waste such as radioactive or chemical waste (Figs 17.1 and 17.2).
1. **Red category (plastic recyclable waste):**
   - Waste generated from tubing, bottles, intravenous tubes and sets, catheter, urine bags, syringe without needles, gloves, etc.
   - These are disposable contaminated waste which can be recyclable.
   - **Waste material is disposed off by autoclaving followed by shredding**.
2. **Yellow category (soiled waste):**
   - It includes:
     - Human anatomical waste such as human tissues, organs, body parts, fetus
     - Animal anatomical waste
     - Soiled waste or items contaminated with blood and/or body fluids, such as dressings, plasters, cotton and bags

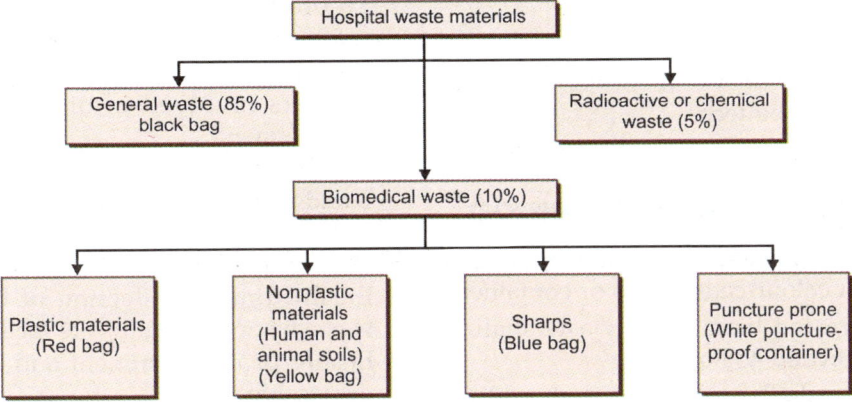

Fig. 17.1: Classification of waste materials

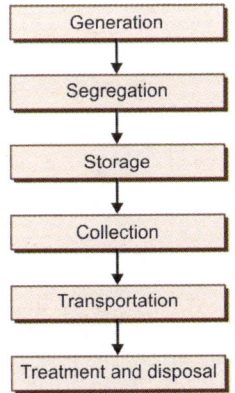

Fig. 17.2: Steps of biomedical waste management

containing residual or discarded blood.

– Expired or discarded medicines

– Cytotoxic drugs and all items contaminated with these drugs

– Linen, mattresses contaminated with blood or body fluid.

– Microbiology, biochemistry and other clinical laboratory waste.

• **Human, animal anatomical waste and soiled waste are disposed off by incineration or plasma pyrolysis or deep burial.**

• Expired medicine and cytotoxic drugs are treated **by incineration**.

• **Laboratory waste is pretreated by non-chlorinated chemicals** as per WHO guidelines.

3. **Blue bags (puncture-proof container):**

• It includes:

– Broken discarded and contaminated glass

– Medicine vials and ampoules except those contaminated with cytotoxic waste.

• Waste materials should be **thoroughly cleaned and then disinfected with sodium hypochloride or by autoclaving.** Finally, it may be **sent for recycling**.

4. **White puncture-proof container:**

• Waste materials include:

– Needles, syringes with needle

– Suture needles, aluminium foils

– Any contaminated sharp objects

• They are **sterilized by autoclaving or by dry heat** before disposal.

5. **Black bags:** They are used for general waste.

6. **Waste not included under biomedical waste rules are:**

- Radioactive waste
- Hazardous chemicals
- Hazardous microorganism
- Lead-acid batteries
- E-waste

SEGREGATION, STORAGE AND TRANSPORT

- Biomedical wastes are segregated in different colour-coded bags or containers.
- No untreated biomedical waste shall be stored beyond 48 hours.
- Occupier shall ensure that it should not produce human health hazards.

Duty of Occupier

- To ensure the segregation of different biomedical waste in respective bags or containers.

- To provide safe, ventilated and secured space for storage of biomedical waste.
- To arrange training for all health care workers involved in biomedical waste management.
- To ensure immunization against hepatitis B and tetanus for workers.

Duty of Operators

- Ensure timely collection of biomedical waste from the health care facilities.
- Ensure proper treatment and disposal of disposable items
- Handing over the recyclable waste after proper treatment.
- Assist health care facility for training of workers.
- Report major accidents and remedial measures.

CHAPTER **18**

Preoperative Assessment, Premedication and Preparation of Patient

Health care provided to a patient before an operation is called preoperative care. It starts as soon as the surgeon takes the decision that operation is necessary for the patient.

Aim of preoperative care is to optimize physical and mental health status of the patient and thus to increase the success of the surgery. Preoperative care also reduces the risk of intraoperative and postoperative complications.

Preoperative care of the patient depends upon the type and duration of surgery, age of the patient and general health of patient.

1. PREOPERATIVE ASSESSMENT

- Enquire the patient about medical history and find out any positive history of major illnesses such as hypertension, diabetes, heart disease, chronic lung disease or neurological problems.
- Record baseline data such as height, weight, temperature, pulse rate, respiratory rate and blood pressure.
- Assist the doctor to carry out a thorough physical examination and to assess the health status of the patient.
- Explain the patient about investigations advised by the doctor and subsequently collect the reports for further evaluations by the doctor.

2. PSYCHOLOGICAL PREPARATION

- Explain the patient about type of surgery, expected duration of surgery and expected duration of hospitalization. Discuss common perioperative problems and their remedies.
- Allow the patient to ask questions and clear all doubts.
- Explain the entire perioperative period in a language, which the patient can understand easily.

3. INFORMED CONSENT

- Before performing a procedure, it is necessary to take permission or consent from the patient. This is particularly important before any invasive or surgical procedure.
- Informed consent means the patient and family members understand the entire perioperative events, including potential risks and complications of both proceeding and nonproceeding of an operative procedure. After proper explanation, permission or consent must be obtained for the entire course of action.
- Obtain consent from the patient/legal guardian (for minor patient)/conservators (for a mentally disabled patient) for each

operation and anaesthesia after explaining the entire procedures.

- Language must be understood by the patient and family members. If necessary, draw pictures to make him understand about the events or use interpreters.
- In case of refusal, written documentation and patient's signature is necessary.

4. PREMEDICATIONS

Choice of premedication depends upon the proposed surgery, type of proposed anaesthesia and, associated medical problems of the patients. Check patient's record file and premedicate strictly as per the advice of anaesthesiologist and surgeon.

Goal of Premedication

- To relieve anxiety
- To ensure good sleep
- To reduce gastric secretions and /or enhance gastric emptying
- To facilitate smooth induction of anaesthesia
- To prevent postoperative nausea and vomiting
- To control infection and antibiotic prophylaxis

Preoperative Advice and Training

- To continue medications as per the advice of doctors for his/her chronic illnesses. Most of the drugs are continued till morning of surgery with sips of water. Certain drugs such as oral contraceptive, oral anticoagulants are stopped as per the advice of the anaesthesiologist.
- Medications for cardiovascular problems are generally continued during preoperative periods. Diuretics are generally withheld on the day of surgery except for thiazide diuretics.
- Antihypertensive medications are generally continued except ACE inhibitors and ARB agents. They are usually withheld 12 to 24 hours prior to surgery.

- Medications for psychiatric and psychological problems should be continued in the preoperative period. Otherwise, exacerbations of symptoms may occur in perioperative period.
- Patients on long-term steroid therapy must take their usual dose on the day of surgery.
- Use of antidiabetic agents depends upon the type of surgery, type of anaesthesia and associated comorbid conditions. Long-acting oral hypoglycaemic agents are withheld on the day of surgery. For major surgical procedure, normoglycaemia is maintained by constant blood sugar level monitoring and infusion of insulin during the perioperative period.
- Stop smoking 4–6 weeks before surgery. It reduces the airway hyper-reactivity and thus reduces the incidence of intraoperative and postoperative complications.
- To encourage deep breathing exercise for prevention of postoperative chest complications.
- To train and assist the patient for using an incentive spirometer. Goal of preoperative incentive spirometry is to improve pulmonary ventilation, facilitate respiratory gaseous exchange and to reduce postoperative respiratory complications.
- **Technique of incentive spirometer:**
  - Hold the spirometer in an upright position
  - Ask the patient to steady the device with one hand and hold the mouthpiece with other hand.
  - Ask the patient to exhale normally and the place lips around the mouthpiece. It should be air-tight.
  - Instruct to take a deep slow inspiration to elevate the balls and then hold the balls 2 seconds initially and gradually increasing to 6 seconds. Nose should be closed during this process.
  - Remove lips from mouthpiece and ask to exhale normally.

- Repeat the same procedure multiple times in a day.
- Training for active and passive exercises of lower limbs to prevent postoperative thrombus formation due to venous stasis.
- Educate the patient about pain relieving measures for postoperative pain.
- To ensure fasting as per preoperative fasting guidelines (Table 18.1).

Table 18.1	Fasting guidelines	
Age of patient	**Fasting time (hour)**	
	Milk and solid	**Clear liquid**
<6 months	4	2
6 months to 3 years	6	2
>3 years	8	2

Skin Preparation for Surgery

- Decontamination of skin to reduce the number of the organism by:
  - Repeated cleaning by antiseptic solutions.
  - Removing hair from proposed surgical site either by wet shaving or by using a depilatory cream.
- Preparation of surgical site depends on the type of surgery;
  - *Head surgery*: Skin preparation for head and neck surgery includes entire head starting from the area above eyebrow up to the back of the neck. On either side, it extends up to ear. Mustache and beard should also be removed in adult male patients.
  - *Chest surgery:* Skin preparation should extend from neck to umbilicus. Laterally it should extend up to midlines anteriorly as well as posteriorly.
  - *Abdominal surgery:* Site preparation extends from axilla to midthigh.
  - *Perineal surgery:* Skin preparation includes the entire perineal region including thigh. Shave pubic hair and inner thigh.
  - *Back surgery:* Prepare entire back; starting from shoulders to knee joints.
  - *Upper limb surgery:* Entire upper limb from axilla to fingertips should be shaved and cleaned with antiseptic solutions.
  - *Lower limb surgery:* Entire lower limb including the area up to umbilicus anteriorly and upper part of buttock posteriorly should be shaved and cleaned with antiseptic solutions.

5. GENERAL PREPARATION

- Remove nail polish, lip stick and make-up, if any.
- Remove jewellery, if any, and hand over to family members.
- Remove contact lenses, dentures, hearing aids, etc.
- Enema and bowel preparation, as per the instructions of surgeon especially before gastrointestinal operations has to be considered.
- Nasogastric tube and urinary catheter insertion as per the instructions of the operating team.

CHAPTER 19

Preoperative Preparation of Operation Room and Transfer of the Patient

GOAL

- To keep the operative room ready for the scheduled operative procedure.
- Ensure complete asepsis.

GENERAL PREPARATIONS

Steps

- Receive a list of operations scheduled for the day.
- Clean and disinfect the operation room including all machines and equipment.
- Ensure availability of adequate sterile instruments for proposed operations.
- Check the scrub room for its readiness with running water, soap and scrubber.
- Ensure uninterrupted power supply and UPS back up.
- Check ceiling light, air conditioning, and OT light for proper functioning.
- Check the functional status of the OT table, diathermy machine and suction apparatus.
- Check central pipe lines, anaesthesia work station, monitors and ventilators to assess the functional status.
- Check emergency medicine and add if any medicine is missing from the tray. Check expiry dates and replace with new medicines at regular intervals.

- Check the functional status of resuscitation equipment including defibrillator.
- Check difficult airway cart
- Based on the proposed surgery, ensure other high-end equipment such as operating microscope, endoscope, laparoscope and C-arm are working properly.
- Collect sterile linen and instrument sets.
- Conduct appropriate trolley layout for different operating procedures enlisted for that day.

INSTRUMENT TROLLEY LAYOUT

Appropriate sterile linen, dressing draping materials and instruments are arranged in a proper order on the designated trolley to perform a particular operation.

Steps

- Person assigned for trolley layout must put on cap, mask, gown and gloves with full aseptic precautions.
- Ensure that the trolley is completely dry. Cover the entire platform of the trolley with sterile waterproof materials (sterile rubber cloth or any other impermeable sterile sheet).
- Take the sterile towel with full aseptic precautions and spread it carefully on the

trolley without touching the unsterile zone. Distal end of the trolley must be draped first than proximal end.

- Open the sterile pack and place it on the trolley.
- Arrange the instruments according to the order of use.
- Discard unnecessary wrappers and foils from the sterile area.
- Cover the trolley with the sterile towel.

TRANSFER THE PATIENT TO PREOPERATIVE ROOM OF OPERATION THEATRE

During Transfer

- Change the dress of the patient and preferably put on a sterile gown.
- Tie an identification card on the arm of the patient where, identification data such as name, age, sex, ward and bed number, diagnosis, operation proposed and hospital registration number should be clearly written. Side of operation (left or right) should be marked with a marker pencil to reduce the chance of confusion.

- Transfer the patients on a trolley and cover the patient with a clean sterile sheet.
- Shift the patient to preoperative room of operation theatre with all relevant documents such as patient record file, X-ray and investigation reports.
- Attendant must accompany throughout the transfer procedure and hand over the patient to nursing personnel of pre-operative room.

Preoperative Room

- Receive patient with patient record file and all investigations report.
- Reconfirm the patient identity, diagnosis, surgery proposed, site of surgery, side of the proposed surgery (left or right, as applicable).
- Check the consent form and blood requisition form. Confirm about the availability of blood.
- Check NPO status.
- Check and record the baseline vital parameters.
- Ensure that preoperative advice has fully complied.

CHAPTER 20

Positioning and Draping of the Patients

Position of the patient on the operation table, preparation of skin and draping of the patients are determined by the proposed operative procedure.

Objectives of Positioning of Surgical Patients

- To optimize the exposure of the surgical site
- To facilitate the intraoperative monitoring of patient
- To minimize the adverse effects associated with the different positions (like the compression of vessels and nerves)
- To ensure the safety of surgical patients

Circulating assistant is primarily responsible for the transfer of the patient and positioning on the operation table. Positioning should be done under the guidance and supervision of the surgeon and anaesthesiologist.

Initially, patient is usually placed in the supine position and covered by a warm cotton blanket. After administration of anaesthesia and permission from anaesthesiologist, the patient may be repositioned for surgery.

If the operation is planned in prone position, then the patient is usually anaesthetized in supine position on transport trolley. After intubation, at least four persons gently lift and turn the patient prone on the operation table.

Precautions during Transfer and Positioning of Patient on Operation Table

- Reconfirm the patient identity.
- Reconfirm the type and site of surgery.
- Lock the transport trolley, operation theatre table, and stabilize the mattresses during transport of the patient from trolley to OT table.
- Assist awake patient during transfer and positioning from both the sides of the table.
- Provide adequate assistance during lifting of unconscious and anaesthesized patient. Movements should be gentle and all protections must be taken to prevent injuries.
- Anaesthesiologist supports the head end of the patient and protects the endotracheal tube during positioning.
- Body exposure should be minimal and thus to prevent hypothermia and preserve dignity.
- During positioning, care must be taken to protect intravenous cannula, catheter, endotracheal tube, etc.
- Arm should not be hyperextended or hyperabducted because it may cause stretching of brachial plexus.
- Pressure points in various positions must be identified and protected by adequate padding.

- Body areas that need adequate padding during positioning are as follows:
  - Supine position—possible pressure points are occiput, heels, elbows and scrotum.
  - Prone position—face especially eyes and ears, knee joints, genitalia and breast.
  - Lateral position—lateral portion of the face including ear, medial knees, axilla, arms, ankles and feet.
- During prone position, the abdomen should be kept free for unobstructed respiratory movements. Towel pad is placed below the thorax and at pelvic region. Minimum four persons are required to position the patient smoothly.
- In supine position, ankles or legs should not be crossed because it may cause pressure on blood vessels or nerves and increases the risk of deep vein thrombosis.
- In lateral position, one pillow must be placed between the two legs to prevent pressure on bony prominences, blood vessels and nerves. Padding should be placed beneath the axilla of the lower side of the body to protect the lower arm from pressure effect caused by body weight.
- During attachments of different accessories to the operation tables, patients must be protected from crush injuries.
- Surface should not create pressure on any parts of the body. If necessary pressure relieving surface may be used, especially in the prolonged surgical procedure (more than two hours).

Complications due to Inappropriate Positioning

- Haemodynamic instability is due to head up or head down position.
- Inadequate ventilation due to thoraco-abdominal compression.
- Tissue damage due to crush injury
- Ischaemia of limbs
- Venous thrombosis
- Peripheral nerve injury

- Optic nerve ischaemia and blindness
- Corneal abrasion

Skin Preparation

The purpose of skin preparation is to make the surgical site as much as possible free from microorganisms, dirt and skin oil and thus to minimize chances of infection from this source.

Skin preparation usually starts at ward and continues till draping of the patient before surgery. Many surgeons advise the patient to take a bath with antimicrobial soap on the day of operation. Body cream, oil or lotion should not be applied after bath. Body piercing jewellery should be removed.

Hair removal can injure the skin and many surgeons do not recommend this procedure. Sometimes hair is very thick, coarse and interferes surgical dressing and draping. Electric clippers are better than shaving razor as they do not damage or injured the skin.

Before Operation

- Take a small table and drape it to create a sterile area.
- Place sterile gloves, two absorbent towels, two-three small bowls for antiseptic solutions, gauze pieces and sponge-holding forceps.
- Pour the antiseptic solution into the bowl.
- Put on gloves.
- Keep two towels at the side of surgical sides to prevent spillage of the excess of antiseptic solutions.
- Hold gauze pieces or sponge with sponge-holding forceps, dip into the antiseptic solution and apply on the surgical site.
- Application of antiseptic solution is done in a circular manner from the incision site to periphery. Solution should not be wiped off; rather it should be allowed to dry up spontaneously.
- Sometimes alcohol is used after drying the antiseptic solution. Alcohol is applied in similar fashion and is allowed to dry before draping.

SPECIFIC ANATOMICAL AREAS

Head and Neck

Eye: Eyelash may be trimmed. The eyelids and periorbital areas are cleaned with a non-irritating antiseptic solution. Conjunctival sac is flushed with non-toxic non-irritant sterile solutions such as normal saline. Take care to prevent spillage of antiseptic solution and to enter in the ear.

Face: Demarcation of the sterile area is difficult, so clean the surrounding area as much as possible. Skin should be cleaned at least up to hairline. Protect ear by putting a cotton ball or gauze. Protect eye by putting a small piece of sterile plastic sheet on it. Clean the nostril with cotton applicators dipped in the antiseptic solution.

Neck: Exposed the area almost up to nipple line and put a sterile towel beyond it. Sterile area should include mandible above, and chest up to nipple line down. Laterally, it should cover from the top of the shoulder up to surgical table line.

Chest and Trunk

Lateral thoracoabdominal area: Expose the surgical site and the adjacent area to be made sterile. Upper arm should be held up during skin preparation. Skin preparation should include chest and abdomen from neck to the iliac crest.

Rectoperitoneal area: Patient is placed in the lithotomy position and a moisture-proof pad is placed below buttocks. Surgical area prepared with antiseptic solution includes pubis, external genitalia, perineum, anus and inner aspect of the thigh.

Scrubbing starts from pubic area gradually goes downward over genitalia and perineum. Take another sponge and clean inner aspect of the thigh. Anus is prepared last.

Vagina: Patient is placed in the lithotomy position and a moisture-proof pad is placed below the buttocks. One sterile towel is placed above the pubis. Cleaning and scrubbing with antiseptic solution start from pubic area gradually moves downward to clean vulva and

perineum. Inner upper third thigh should be cleaned with the antiseptic solution. The vagina and cervix should be cleaned with separate sponges in sponge-holding forceps.

Extremities: A moisture-proof sterile draping material is placed on the table beneath the extremity to be operated. It is normally removed, once skin preparation is over. Extremity is held at the distal part (foot or hand) by a person wearing sterile gloves. Full circumference of the extremity is prepared with the antiseptic solution and makes the area sterile.

DRAPING

Draping is a process of covering the surrounding area of the surgical site with a sterile material to create an adequate sterile field for operation.

Draping materials may be a self-adhesive sheet, non-woven synthetic disposable sheet or reusable textile fabrics sheet. Draping materials may be a simple towel or fenestrated sheets (opening within the sheet to incision site).

Basic Principles of Draping

- Place the sterile draping materials on the dry sterile trolley. Handle the draping materials as less as possible.
- After skin preparation, sufficient time should be given to dry the antiseptic solution.
- Never go across the operation table to drape the opposite side.
- Take the towel and towel clip (if necessary) and hold it at the side of the table from where surgeon is going to apply it.
- Hold the draping material high enough to avoid touching the unsterile area.
- Keep the draping material high and gradually bring over the surgical field. Once it reaches the proper place, lay it down on the surgical site.
- Once draping material is placed, it should not move or adjust further.
- If during this process, sterile draping material gets contaminated, discard it without contaminating other items.

CHAPTER 21

Role of the Scrub Assistant

Scrub assistant is a specially trained person who works with surgeons and other surgical team members in the operating room. A scrub assistant supplies the instruments to the surgeon throughout the surgical procedure, keeps an eye on operative field and silently assists the surgical team.

- Scrub assistants should be in OT attire with cap and mask same as other team members. Then they should wear sterile gown and gloves after proper scrubbing.
- Scrub assistants should have basic knowledge of surgical steps. They should have full knowledge of instruments and operation theatre equipment.

ROLE OF THE SCRUB ASSISTANT

- **Preparation before the surgical procedure:**
  - Work with circulating assistant to prepare operation room for proposed surgery.
  - Acquire knowledge about surgical procedure; enquire about any specific need for the proposed procedure.
  - Discuss with the surgical team about the key points of surgery and ask for any specific needs of surgical team.
  - Ensure about adequate availability of disposables, suture materials, implants, etc.

- **Maintenance of sterility:**
  - Scrubbing, gowning and gloving before entering the sterile zone.
  - To establish and maintain the sterile field.
  - To assist the surgical team and facilitate the surgical procedure.
  - Anticipate the needs of sterile team and prepare to respond immediately.

- **Adaptability to fulfill the need of surgical team:**
  - Participate in pre-incision time out with the entire surgical team
  - Take appropriate measures to maintain a sterile area throughout the surgical procedure.
  - Take remedial measures, if there is any breach of sterile technique.
  - Ensure the uninterrupted supply of materials as per the requirement of the surgeon.
  - Maintain instrument trolley neat and in order for easy and uninterrupted supply of instruments to the surgical team.

- **Ensure accountability:**
  - Record baseline counts with circulating assistant.
  - Receive specimen and hand over to circulating assistant.

– Draw medication and report the volume of medicine used.
– Recheck the counts of instruments, suture materials, mops and disposables.
– Return the unutilized implants.

• **Ensure safety of patient:**
– Check and recheck the counts of various items with circulating assistant.
– Prevention of unsterile objects within the surgical site of patient.
– Protect from sharp objects and prevent injury.

STEPS OF ACTIVITIES OF SCRUB ASSISTANT

• **Plan for operation room set up along with circulating assistant:**
– Plan for correct position of the operation table.
– Plan for position of anaesthesia machine, monitors and anaesthesiologist.
– Plan for position of instrument tables in relation to the surgical field.
– Ensure clean path for transport of patient without hampering the sterility of operation theatre.
– Ensure clear path for emergency equipment to deal any emergency.

• **Jointly work with circulating assistant and ensure availability of surgical instruments, disposables and draping materials:**
– Check instrument sets, ensure sterility and check the integrity of packets.
– Ensure adequate supply of draping materials and sterile towels.
– Ensure availability of different types of suture materials in various sizes, staplers, sponges, mops, dressing materials, drainage tubes, etc.

• **Prepare to enter sterile zone:**
– Open gown and gloves for self-use.
– Wash and clean hand up to elbow joint with soap water under running water.

– Put on gown and gloves using closed glove procedure.

• **Set up instrument trolley:**
– Ensure that instrument trolley is clean and dry. Put a sterile waterproof cover over it.
– Receive sterile towel from circulating assistant spread over the table carefully without touching the unsterile area.
– Drape distal part of trolley first then proximal end.
– Receive sterile pack from circulating assistant and keep instrument tray and instruments gently on the instrument trolley.
– Arrange instrument neatly and according to the order of use.
– Discard unnecessary wrappers and foils from the sterile field.
– Cover the trolley with a sterile towel till surgeon is ready to start the surgery.
– Drape Mayo stand with sterile waterproof materials and arrange instruments.

• **To assist surgical team during gowning and gloving:**
– Assist surgical team to glove and gown using open-assisted or closed-assisted methods.
– Change of contaminated gloves using open method.

• **Patient positioning:**
– Scrub assistant should stand away and remain sterile during the positioning of the patient. Remember positioning is an unsterile activity.
– Expose operative site while adequately cover other areas by circulating assistants.

• **Cleaning with bactericidal solution and draping of patient:**
– Assist surgeon to clean the site with a bactericidal solution.

– Offer sterile towels and towel clips to surgeon and assistant during draping of the operative site.

– Assist surgeon to apply 'impermeable sterile adhesive' evenly without any air pockets.

• **Start of operative procedure:**

– Participate in time out process before supplying skin scalpel to surgeon as a member of the surgical team.

– Supply two sponges on the surgical field adjacent to the incision.

– Provide scalpel to the main surgeon for skin incision.

– Supply diathermy pencil tip to achieve haemostasis.

– Clean the diathermy pencil tip time to time.

– Keep an eye on operative field and supply instruments, sponges, suture materials step by step as per the necessity of surgical procedure.

– Receive specimens from surgeon and hand over to circulating assistant for labelling and early transport to respective laboratory.

– Count sponges, instruments especially sharp materials at each cavity before cavity closure.

– Perform closing counts of sponges, instruments and sharp materials with circulating assistant during surgical site closure.

– Open soiled sponges before discarding into sponge bucket.

• **Activity during postoperative dressings and drainage:**

– Following closure of incision by surgeon, area should be cleaned by a wet sponge followed by dry sponge and made area dry.

– Place dressing materials over the surgical site after cleaning the incision site.

– Disconnect tubing and cords and remove draping materials.

– Skin surrounding the dressing materials should be cleaned and dried.

– Fix the dressing materials with transparent adhesive tape.

• **Activity at the end of the surgical procedure:**

– All reusable instruments should be disassembled and then place on a container for cleaning and decontamination.

– Disarm scalpels and dispose sharp materials on sharps container.

– Dispose biologic trash in biohazard containers.

– Dispose clean trash in a regular garbage container.

– Remove contaminated gown first then remove gloves.

– Wash hands with soap and water.

– Clean all reusable instruments with running water followed by antiseptic solution.

– Use antiseptic solution to clean all equipment used during surgery.

– Prepare operation theatre for the next operation.

CHAPTER 22

Role of the Circulating Assistant

Circulating assistant of an operation theatre is a person, who prepares operation room before operation, continuously monitors and supports the patients and surgical team without disturbing the sterile area, records the progress of operation, counts instruments at the end of the operation and preserves specimens, if any.

- In operation room, there are two distinct areas—sterile operating field and the non-sterile area.
- Circulating assistant remains in non-sterile area and supports the operating team from outside.
- Since circulating assistant works in non-sterile field, it is not necessary to scrub like other members of the operative team who are directly involved in the act of surgical procedure.
- However, the circulating assistant should wear sterile dress, cap and mask and take appropriate measures to maintain clean conditions within operation theatre.

ROLE OF CIRCULATING ASSISTANT

- **General preparation:**
  - Clean and disinfect operation room including machines and equipment used during the operation.
  - Check all equipment and reconfirm their functional status
  - Open sterile supplies.
- **Patient care:**
  - Check patient identifications, check the type of surgery and site of surgery.
  - Check preoperative vital parameters: Pulse, blood pressure, temperature, oxygen saturation, etc.
  - Transfer the patient from trolley to the operation table.
  - Participate in preoperative time out procedure.
  - Assist anaesthesiologist during induction of anaesthesia and provide necessary support during the entire course of anaesthesia.
  - Provide skin antisepsis before scrub team conduct thorough cleaning, antisepsis and draping.
  - Provide adequate attention to intra-operative heat loss of patient specially neonate for prevention of hypothermia.
  - Provide attention to prevent electro-surgical injury while putting the diathermy plate.
  - Supply suture materials, mops, or any other items to scrub assistant as per the demand of the surgical team.

- **Intraoperative coordination with other team members:**
  - Assist each member of sterile team during scrubbing, gowning, gloving and provide free passage to enter in the sterile area.
  - Assist during positioning, preparing and draping the patient and surgical field.
  - Connect surgical machinery.
  - Emergency response to patient care.
  - Communications with other persons for any emergency needs.

- **Anticipations:**
  - Steps of proposed surgical procedure
  - Requirements of surgical team
  - Anticipations and protections of sterile team from exposure to radiation
  - Potential changes in patient physiological condition as per associated co-morbid conditions, if any.

- **Responsibilities:**
  - Participate in time out as a member of surgical team.
  - Documentations related to patient parameters, details of instruments, sutures and implants.
  - Collection, preservation and hand over of specimens for early transport to the respective laboratory.
  - Accountability for instruments, mops, sponges, disposables and implants, if any.
  - Transport of patient from operation theatre to post-anaesthesia care unit and hand over of patient.

STEPS OF ACTIVITIES OF CIRCULATING ASSISTANT

- **Set-up operation room:**
  - Plan for correct position of the operation table.
  - Plan for position of anaesthesia machine, monitor and anaesthesiologist.
  - Plan for position of instrument tables in relation to the surgical field.

  - Ensure clean path for transport of patient without hampering the sterility of operation theatre.
  - Ensure clear path for emergency equipment to deal any emergency.

- **Ensure availability of standard operation theatre equipment:**
  - Appropriate operation theatre table including arm boards. Ensure the movements and different tilts of the table are feasible either manually or electronically.
  - Two IV poles
  - Check availability of Mayo stands and instrument tables.
  - Check OT light, suction apparatus and diathermy and ensure their functional status.
  - Check all anaesthesia and surgery related equipment and confirm their functional status.
  - Check availability of platform steps for the surgical team.

- **Ensure availability of surgical instruments, disposables and draping material as per requirement of proposed surgical procedure:**
  - Check instrument sets, ensure sterility and check the integrity of packets.
  - Ensure adequate supply of draping materials and sterile towels.
  - Ensure the availability of following items:
    - Different types of suture materials in various sizes
    - Staplers
    - Sponges and/or mops
    - Dressing materials
    - Drainage tubes

- **Set-up instrument table:**
  - Place sterile packed surgical instrument sets on the clean, dry and sterile surface of instrument table.
  - Coordinate with scrub assistant for count and documentation of instruments displayed in the instrument table.

– Provide adequate gowns and gloves on another sterile table for surgeon and assistants. Assist them during gowning and gloving. Tie gowns of surgical team at the back.

• **Supply antiseptic solutions:**
– Obtain antiseptic solutions for establishing a sterile area.
– Validate the type of antiseptic solution, its concentration and dose jointly with scrub assistant.

• **Transfer the patient to the operation table:**
– Reconfirm patient identity, site and type of surgery.
– Check NPO (nothing per mouth) status. –Check the preoperative order and confirm the implementation of same.
– Hand over patient record sheets including X-rays, scans and other relevant diagnostic reports.

• **Assist anaesthesiologist:**
– Assist for positioning of the patient during regional anaesthesia.
– Assist anaesthesiologist during induction of general anaesthesia.
  ▪ Assist to establish IV cannulation.
  ▪ Assist during intubation by applying cricoid pressure.
– Assist in perioperative monitoring, administration of drugs, IV fluids, etc.
– Assist during reversal of anaesthesia and recovery.

• **Patient positioning, skin preparation and draping:**
– Wait until anaesthesiologist is sure about the safety of patient for positioning.
– Position the patient according to the type of surgical procedure under the supervision of surgeon and anaesthesiologist.
– Ensure adequate exposure of surgical site.
– Apply diathermy plates in an appropriate location.
– Supply adequate antiseptic solutions and draping materials to scrub assistant for preparing absolutely sterile area for surgery.

• **Position of instruments trolley, surgical team and intraoperative supports:**
– Assist scrub person to move sterile table adjacent to the surgical field.
– Attach cables, tubing to respective devices.
– Initiate time out, verify patient name, procedure and correct site.
– Carefully monitor intraoperative events and supply, if any requirement from the surgical team.
– Receive specimen, preserve it and hand over for early transport.
– Communicate with family as per the instructions of the surgical team during surgery.

• **Dressing and drains:**
– Ensure proper drainage from drainage tube.
– Supply adequate dressing materials to scrub assistant to apply on the surgical field at the end of the procedure.
– Fix dressing materials with adhesive tape. Avoid affixing to hairy surface.

• **Post-procedural activities:**
– Reconfirm closing count with scrub assistant. It includes instruments, implants, mops, sponges, suture materials or any other items present in the surgical field.
– Prepare hand-off notes for hand over to post-anaesthesia care unit. It includes:
  ▪ Patient's name, age, hospital registration number
  ▪ Allergies/sensitivities, if any
  ▪ Current procedure and type of anaesthesia
  ▪ Details of family member or contact person
  ▪ Any important intraoperative events
  ▪ Any patient comorbidity.
– Transport patient to post-anaesthesia care unit with anaesthesia provider.

CHAPTER 23

Intraoperative Monitoring of Patients

Administration of anaesthesia is associated with changes in the internal homeostasis, especially in cardiovascular, respiratory and central nervous systems. Therefore, constant monitoring is necessary for the well-being of patients.

During intraoperative period, monitoring of the patient is done by the following ways.

- Clinical monitoring
- Instrumental monitoring
  - Noninvasive monitoring
  - Invasive monitoring

CLINICAL MONITORING

The most important factor for clinical monitoring is the continuous presence of a competent anaesthesiologist. The anaesthesiologist is totally responsible for the patients, whether surgery is conducted under general anaesthesia, regional anaesthesia or sedation with multiple drugs.

Following clinical parameters should be monitored during surgery.

- *Circulation:*
  - Pulse rate, rhythm, volume
  - Skin elasticity
  - Temperature
  - Urine output (if catheterized)

- *Respiration:*
  - In patients with spontaneous ventilation
    - Tidal volume
    - Respiratory rate
    - Any signs of airway obstruction
  - In paralyzed patients with controlled ventilation
    - Feeling of the reservoir bag
    - Respiratory efforts

- *Oxygenation:* Colour of the blood, skin and mucous membrane

- *Depth of anaesthesia:*
  - Presence or absence of lacrimation
  - Presence or absence of sweating
  - Muscle movements
  - Size of pupils

INSTRUMENTAL MONITORING

Noninvasive Monitoring

- Extent of monitoring depends upon the preoperative condition of the patient, type of anaesthesia, type and duration of surgery.
- Minimum monitoring standards (as per Indian Society of Anaesthesiologist guidelines) include:
  - Noninvasive blood pressure

93

- Electrocardiograph (ECG)
- Pulse oximetry
- Capnography although is not mandatory but very important in the perioperative period.
- Monitoring of body temperature, neuromuscular blockade and depth of anaesthesia is desirable.
- Commonly heart rate, rhythm, blood pressure, ECG and oxygen saturation is continuously monitored during the perioperative period by a multimodular monitoring system (Fig. 23.1).

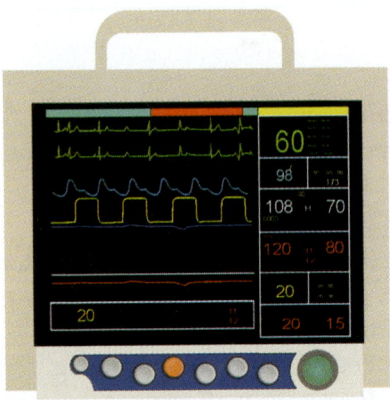

Fig. 23.1: Multimodular monitoring system

Electrocardiograph (ECG)

- Electrocardiograph is a surface reflection of depolarizing and nondepolarizing electrical activity of various parts of the heart.
- ECG electrodes are placed on the chest or limbs of the patient to detect the electrical activity of the heart. It is boosted by an amplifier. An oscilloscope finally displays the amplified ECG signal.
- ECG is used to monitor heart rate, presence of any dysrhythmia and pacemaker's function. It also detects the presence of myocardial ischaemia.
- Lead II is monitored commonly for identifying arrhythmias. Lead V_5 should be monitored continuously especially in patient with ischaemic heart disease.

- Any change in ECG must be confirmed by a 12-lead ECG.

Noninvasive Blood Pressure Monitor (NIBP)

- NIBP monitor consists of compression cuff with a microprocessor and digital display device. Compression cuff is wrapped around a limb, usually upper arm and inflated above the systolic pressure.
- Width of the cuff should be 40% of the mid-circumference of the limb and length should be twice the width.
- Automated device used for blood pressure monitoring by a noninvasive method is based on oscillotonometric technique.
- The microprocessor is set to control the sequence of inflation and deflation.
- Cuff is inflated above the systolic pressure to stop the flow of blood through artery and then slowly deflated.
- Return of blood flow causes oscillation in the cuff pressure and is interpreted by the microprocessor as systolic blood pressure.
- The mean arterial pressure corresponds to the maximum oscillation and the diastolic pressure corresponds to rapidly decreasing oscillation.
- These signals are digitalized, filtered and electronically processed to display systolic, mean and diastolic blood pressure.

Pulse Oximetry

- The pulse oximetry displays real-time oxygen saturation of haemoglobin continuously by noninvasive technique.
- Pulse oximeter works on the principle of Beer-Lambert law. According to this law, the amount of light absorbed by a solution is directly proportional to the amount of solute in it (Fig. 23.2).
- Various concentrations of oxyhaemoglobin and reduced haemoglobin at arterial blood, differential absorption of light by them and arterial pulsation are utilized in the construction of pulse oximeter.

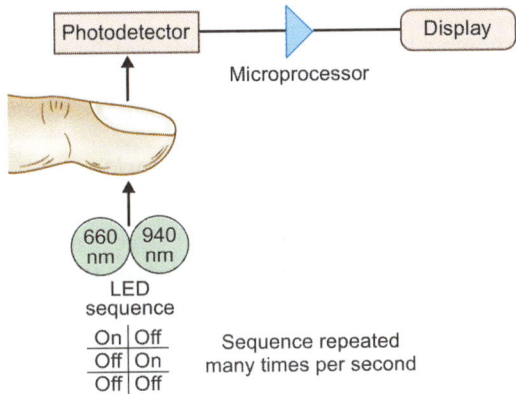

Fig. 23.2: Working principle of the pulse oximeter

- The pulse oximeter probe consists of a light source one side, that delivers both red (660 nm) and infrared (940 nm) light. One photodetector is present on the other side to detect the amount of light absorbed by oxy and reduced haemoglobin. The probe is placed on the finger, toe or ear lobe.
- Oxyhaemoglobin absorbs more light at 940 nm and reduced haemoglobin absorbs more light at 660 nm.
- Light source emits alternately red and infrared light separately by a gap, at a frequency of 400 Hz. In these wavelengths, absorption spectra of reduced and oxygenated haemoglobin are widely separated and nearly equal.
- Pulse oximeter discriminates between arterial blood and other tissue due to its pulsatile nature, causing constant change in the transmitted light. Total amount of haemoglobin and proportion of oxyhaemoglobin is determined.
- Software calculates the arterial oxygen saturation from absorption data.

Significance

- Normal oxygen saturation of a healthy person is 98–100%.
- If saturation is 90%, hypoxia is imminent. It corresponds to PaO_2 of 60 mm Hg.

Limitations

- Any movement in the parts of the body connected to the pulse oximetry probe causes irregular reading.
- Hypothermia, low perfusion, nail polish may cause oxygen saturation reading unreliable or unpredictable.
- Carboxyhaemoglobin, methaemoglobin or use of certain dye make pulse oximeter reading unreliable and wrong.

Capnograph

- Capnograph (Fig. 23.3) means measurement and graphically display of carbon dioxide concentration throughout the respiratory cycle.
- Carbon dioxide present in the respiratory gases absorbs infrared light in proportion to its concentrations. In this way, the amount of CO_2 present in a mixture is measured.
- When carbon dioxide concentration is displayed against time, a capnograph is obtained. Capnograph consists of four phases.
  – Phase I: Inspiratory baseline (dead space gases)
  – Phase II: Expiratory upstroke (mixed alveolar and dead space gases)
  – Phase III: Expiratory plateau (alveolar gases)
  – Phase IV: Inspiratory downstroke (inspiratory gases)

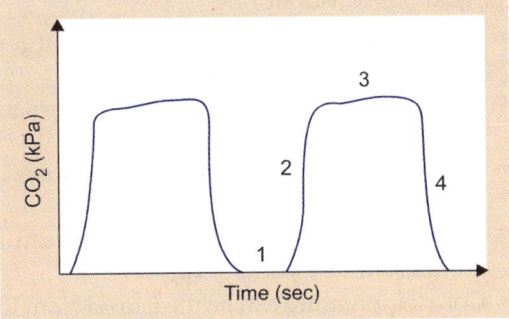

Fig. 23.3: Normal capnograph

- The carbon dioxide concentration at the end of expiration is called end-tidal carbon dioxide. Normal range is 35–40 mm Hg. It is 2–5 mm Hg less than arterial CO_2 pressure.

Uses

- End-tidal carbon dioxide level may be increased or decreased in different pathological conditions.
- End-tidal carbon dioxide zero indicates oesophageal intubation, accidental extubation, disconnection or cardiac arrest.
- If the end tidal carbon dioxide level is more than 15 mm Hg, during resuscitation following cardiac arrest, chances of recovery is higher.

Neuromuscular Monitoring

- It is used to assess the degree of neuromuscular block following use of neuromuscular blocking agents or muscle relaxant.
- A supramaximal electrical stimulus between 10 and 50 mA is applied to a superficial peripheral motor nerve such as ulnar nerve and the response of muscles supplied by such nerve is assessed.
- Stimulus may be given as a single stimulus, train of four stimulus, tetanic stimulus or double-burst stimulus.
- Muscle response is observed following a stimulus delivered to the nerve. Depending upon the muscular response, the degree of the neuromuscular block can be analyzed.

Temperature Monitoring

- Monitoring of temperature during surgery is a common and routine procedure.
- Different types of thermometer probes are used for intraoperative monitoring.
- They can be thermisters, thermocouples or infrared thermometers.
- Core, as well as surface or skin temperature are measured during surgery.
- Core temperature can be measured from the rectum, oesophagus, tympanic membrane or bladder.

Invasive Monitoring

Invasive monitoring of cardiovascular system is sometime required in many major cardiovascular or neurosurgical operations.

Direct Arterial Pressure Monitoring

Direct arterial pressure monitor displays continuous real-time arterial waveform and detects beat-to-beat variations in blood pressure.

Indications

- Critically ill patients
- Patients with unstable or compromised cardiovascular system
- Cardiopulmonary bypass
- Surgical procedure where hypotensive anaesthesia is indicated.

Procedure

- Radial artery is usually cannulated by 20G or 22G cannula. Sometimes dorsalis pedis and femoral arteries are also used.
- Arterial cannula is connected to the pressure transducer through a fluid-filled catheter. The pressure transducer consists of a diaphragm which separates connecting catheter and electronic measuring system. Diaphragm contains four strain gauges which converts mechanical movement of the diaphragm into electrical signals.
- To minimize the error, system must be calibrated, levelled and made it zero at the level of the heart.

Information obtained from invasive blood pressure monitoring:

- Beat-to-beat monitoring of systolic, mean and diastolic blood pressure.
- Monitoring heart rate and rhythm.
- **Contractility:** If contractility of heart is good, then upstroke of the arterial waveform will be steep.
- **Preload:** Variations in systolic blood pressure of more than 10% in different phases of respiration indicate hypovolaemia.

Central Venous Pressure Monitoring

- Catheter is inserted into central vein and the tip is positioned in the superior vena cava. It measures the pressure of the right atrium or central venous pressure.

- Central venous catheter is connected to a pressure transducer, which converts mechanical movements into electronic signals. Electronic signals finally display as waveform and determine the numerical value of central venous pressure.

- Normal central venous pressure is 2–5 cm H_2O.

- For central venous cannulation, right internal jugular vein or subclavian vein is preferred.

Indications

- To measure central venous pressure
- To guide fluid therapy
- For parenteral nutrition
- For administration of drugs such as chemotherapeutic agents, vasopressors, etc.

CHAPTER 24

Post-Anaesthesia Care of Patients

At the end of any surgical procedure, anaesthetic agents are discontinued to recover the patient from the effects of anaesthesia. Recovery from anaesthesia and surgery may be associated with a number of physiological disturbances that may affect multiple vital organs. Therefore, to optimize the care immediately after surgery, it is desirable to transfer the patient in post-anaesthesia care unit (PACU).

The post-anaesthesia care unit is designed to provide close monitoring and care to a patient during the transition period, i.e. recovering from anaesthesia or sedation to a fully awake state.

GENERAL GUIDELINES OF POST-ANAESTHESIA CARE

- All patients received general anaesthesia or regional anaesthesia should receive appropriate post-anaesthesia care.
- Patient should be continuously monitored and treated during transport from the operation table to post-anaesthesia care unit (PACU) by an anaesthesiologist.
- On arrival at PACU, the patient should be re-evaluated. All relevant information including written instructions should be handed over to the responsible health care provider of post-anaesthesia care unit.

- Patient should be evaluated continuously in PACU. Particular attention should be given to oxygenation, ventilation and circulation.
- Vital signs should be recorded at least at an interval of 15 minutes. It should be done more frequently in critically ill patients. Any abnormal finding should be reported to on-duty physician for further assessment and management.
- On-duty physician is responsible for the discharge of the patient from post-anaesthesia care unit.

MONITORING OF PATIENT IN PACU

- **Respiration:**
  - Assessment for airway patency
  - Respiratory rate
  - Oxygen saturation
- **Cardiovascular:**
  - Heart rate and/or pulse rate
  - Blood pressure
  - ECG monitoring should be available for immediate use.
- **Neurological:**
  - Patient must be assessed periodically for mental alertness.

- If the patient receives sedative or narcotic as per the postoperative direction, it should be documented.
- **Neuromuscular:** If the patient has received neuromuscular blocking agent during anaesthesia, then muscle power should be checked in the immediate postoperative period by checking hand grip or ability to raise head for at least 5 seconds.
- Temperature should be monitored at regular intervals.
- Hydration status, urine output, drainage and bleeding from the surgical site should be checked at regular intervals.
- Patient should be assessed for post-operative pain and nausea and vomiting. Appropriate measures should be taken as per the advice of anaesthesiologist.
- Follow the written instructions given by the surgical team without alteration.
- Inform on-duty physician or anaesthesiologist, if there is any warning sign noticed during monitoring.

GENERAL CARE OF POSTOPERATIVE PATIENTS

Oxygen Therapy

Transient hypoxemia is not uncommon even in healthy patients during the immediate postoperative period. Therefore, all patients recovering from general anaesthesia must be monitored by pulse oximetry and should receive supplemental oxygen.

- Choice of oxygen delivery system depends upon the degree of hypoxaemia, type of surgical procedure and pre-existing patient comorbidities.
- Oxygen therapy through a traditional nasal cannula with bubble humidifier can increase FiO_2 up to 0.44.
- Higher FiO_2 can be delivered by facemask with the non-rebreathing system.
- Oxygen therapy should be carefully controlled in patients with a history of CO_2 retention or hypercapnia, such as asthma and COPD patients.

Prevention of Postoperative Nausea and Vomiting

- Postoperative nausea and vomiting (PONV) is common and affects ≥30% of all surgical patients.
- PONV is not only distressful for patients but may:
  - Delay discharge from the recovery room
  - Cause electrolyte imbalance.
- The causes of postoperative nausea and vomiting are multifactorial and PONV has an association with certain anaesthetic agents, type of surgical procedure and patients' intrinsic factors such as the history of motion sickness.
- Prophylaxis antiemetic is recommended in those patients, who are prone to develop PONV.
- Nausea and vomiting should be recorded and reported to on-duty physician for further management.

Management of Postoperative Pain

- Pain is one of the inevitable side effects of surgery. Anaesthesiologist takes various measures to alleviate postoperative pain.
- Assess the severity of pain by using any pain measuring tool.
- Visual Analog Scale is the most commonly used tool for detection of severity of pain. Scale consists of 0 at one end and 10 at another end. Zero means no pain and 10 mean worst possible pains. The patient is asked to express the severity of pain by placing the finger at a particular point between these two extremes of visual analog scale. VAS ≥4 is considered as significant pain.

0 ————————————— 10

Visual Analog Scale

- Follow the instructions of anaesthesiologist for management of postoperative pain. Pain relief is achieved by systemic analgesics/narcotics, local infiltration of surgical incision by local anaesthetic agents, nerve blocks, plexus block, central neuraxial block or combinations of them.
- If pain is still unbearable, on-duty physician should be reported for further management.

Prevention and Management of Shivering

- Shivering is usually due to hypothermia which is very common in elderly and paediatric patients. Hypothermia is commonly observed following prolonged surgery or intravenous infusion of a large volume of cold fluids. Shivering is also common after the use of certain anaesthetic agents.
- Shivering is not only distressful for the patient but also increases the metabolism of the patient. It may increase oxygen consumptions by 300–500%.
- Hypothermia should be prevented by using warming devices like warming blankets and infusion of warm intravenous solutions.
- Oxygen supplementation should be done because shivering increases the metabolic rate and oxygen consumption.
- Pharmacological interventions such as small doses of pethidine or clonidine may be required to control the postoperative shivering. On-duty physician should be called for such management.

CHAPTER 25

Discharge from Post-Anaesthesia Care Unit

Postoperative patients may be transferred from post-anaesthesia care unit (PACU) to phase 2 recoveries, surgical ward or directly to the home. Therefore, criteria for discharge may differ according to quality of postoperative assessment and care is feasible in the proposed place of shifting.

Ideally, all patients should be assessed by an anaesthesiologist, before they are declared fit to discharge from post-anaesthesia care unit. However, other health care provider such as PACU nurse may take the decision regarding discharge from PACU, if patient fulfills all the discharging criteria approved by the department of anaesthesia.

MINIMUM DISCHARGE CRITERIA

- Easy arousability
- Full orientation
- Ability to maintain and protect the airway.
- Stable vital signs for at least 30 minutes.
- No surgical complications such as active bleeding.
- Ability to call for help, if necessary.
- Received last dose of the parental opioid, at least 30 minutes before discharge.
- No or minimum pain.
- Minimum postoperative nausea vomiting.

POST-ANAESTHESIA SCORING SYSTEM

A number of scoring systems have been developed to assess and to take the decision regarding the transfer of the patient from PACU. By these post-anaesthesia scoring systems, it is easy to assess the fitness of the patient for discharge by health care providers such as recovery nurses.

Post-Anaesthesia Aldrete Recovery Score
(Table 25.1)

- A score of 9 out of 10 is considered adequate for discharge from the PACU.
- Patient received regional anaesthesia should be assessed for recovery from sensory and motor blockade. Complete recovery from regional anaesthesia prevents inadvertent injuries due to motor weakness or sensory deficit.
- Patients should have minimum post-operative pain and nausea and vomiting.

DISCHARGE OF OUT-PATIENTS

- Apart from the monitoring of regular vital parameters to assess the fitness of the patient for discharge from PACU, patients treated as day care surgery are also assessed for home readiness and complete psycho-motor recovery.

Table 25.1	Post-anaesthesia Aldrete recovery scores	
Variable		**Score**
Activity		
Able to move four extremities on command		2
Able to move two extremities on command		1
Able to move no extremity on command		0
Breathing		
Able to breathe deeply and cough freely		2
Dyspnoea, shallow or limited breathing		1
Apnoea		0
Circulation		
Systemic blood pressure ≤20 of preanaesthetic level		2
Systemic blood pressure is 20 to 50% of the preanaesthetic level		1
Systemic blood pressure is ≥50% of the preanaesthetic level		0
Consciousness		
Fully awake		2
Arousable		1
Not responding		0
Oxygen saturation		
>92% while breathing room air		2
Needs supplemental oxygen to maintain oxygen saturation >90%		1
Oxygen saturation <90% with supplemental oxygen		0

- Patients received regional anaesthesia should also be assessed for recovery of proprioception, sympathetic tone, bladder function and motor strength.
- Urination, drinking or eating before discharge is no longer required except in patient with a history of urinary retention and diabetes.

Post-Anaesthesia Discharge Scoring System (PADS) for Release Home to a Responsible Adult

- All patients following day care surgery must be discharged in the presence of a responsible adult who will take care of the patient at home.
- Facility to contact medical centre should be available, if there is any adverse effect or complication after discharge following day care surgery. Effective transport facility such as ambulance service should be easily available, if the patient needs hospitalization (Table 25.2).

Table 25.2	Post-anaesthesia discharge scoring system (PADS)	
Variable		**Score**
Vital signs (stable and consistent with age and preanaesthetic baseline)		
Systemic blood pressure and heart rate within 20% of the preanaesthetic level		2
Systemic blood pressure and heart rate 20 to 40% of the preanaesthetic level		1
Systemic blood pressure and heart rate >40% of the preanaesthetic levem		0
Activity level (able to ambulate at preoperative level)		
Steady gait without dizziness or recovery to achieve preanaesthetic status		2
Ambulation possible with assistance		1
Unable to ambulate		0
Nausea and vomiting		
None		2
Moderate		1
Severe		0
Pain (minimal to no pain, controllable with oral analgesics) acceptability		
Yes		2
No		1
Surgical bleeding (consistence with that expected for the surgical procedure)		
Minimal (no dressing change)		2
Moderate (1–2 dressing change required)		1
Severe (≥3 dressing change required)		0

- A score of 9 out of 10 is considered adequate for discharge and ready to release for home.
- Patients should not be allowed to drive or return to work for at least 24 to 72 hours or till there is complete psychomotor recovery.
- In the day care surgery set-up, postoperative pain is the most significant cause of the delayed discharge and unplanned hospital admission. Intense prophylactic analgesic therapy may be beneficial in this scenario.

CHAPTER **26**

Common General Surgery

Laparotomy

It is a surgical procedure to open the abdomen, to visualize the abdominal organs and to explore uncertain abdominal pathology. In traditional laparotomy, a large incision is made on the abdominal wall to see the cavity. After identifying the actual pathology in the organ, necessary operations are performed. For example, splenectomy is done for rupture of the spleen and appendectomy is done for appendicitis. The position of the patient on the table is usually supine.

In instrument trolley, following instruments must be kept ready for laparotomy.

- Towel clips
- Surgical blade with handle
- Non-toothed forceps
- Toothed forceps
- Scissors
- Sponge-holding forceps
- Allis forceps
- Artery forceps
- Babcock's tissue forceps
- Deaver's retractor
- Langenbeck retractor
- Curved round body needle
- Curved/straight cutting needle
- Needle holder
- Corrugated rubber drain
- Different suture material
- Swabs/gauze piece

Appendicectomy

The appendix is a part of gastrointestinal tract located near ileocaecal junction. Appendicectomy is a surgical procedure where appendix is removed. The operation is done in supine position of the patient. After opening the abdomen, the appendix is identified and holds with Babcock's tissue-holding forceps. The appendix is removed, and the stump is cauterized with spirit or carbolic acid or saline. The abdomen is closed in layers.

Instruments: Same set of instruments as required for laparotomy.

Cholecystectomy

Surgical removal of the gallbladder is called cholecystectomy. It is done in cases with gallstone, cholecystitis, empyema gallbladder and mucocoele gallbladder. Cholecystectomy can be done by open approach or by laparoscope.

Open Cholecystectomy

After opening the abdomen, the colon is pushed downward and stomach medially to indentify the gallbladder. It is separated from the liver bed. Cystic artery and cystic duct are identified and ligated. A drain is placed, which is usually removed after 72 hours.

Instruments: Apart from the instruments required for laparotomy, the following should be added to the instrument trolley.

- CBD retractors
- Gallstone-holding forceps
- Gallstone probe
- T-tube

Laparoscopic Cholecystectomy

It is the most popular method for the removal of gallbladder. Gas is introduced within the abdominal cavity to create space for operation. Four small incisions are given on following points to introduce telescope and working channel.

- One at umbilicus
- One at the midline of epigastrium
- Two at the midclavicular and anterior axillary line at subcostal region.

Instrument: Laparoscope with all accessories.

Position of the patient: Head up position.

Cholecystostomy

Cholecystostomy is an operation where an opening in the gallbladder is made to remove gallstones, to drain empyema or for any other purposes. Exposure of gallbladder is same as done in cholecystectomy operation.

Position of patient: Supine position on the table.

Instruments: Same as required for cholecystectomy and one Foley catheter.

Gastrojejunostomy

Gastrojejunostomy is a surgical procedure where an anastomosis between the stomach and jejunum is done to create a bypass for content of the stomach.

Position of the patient: Supine on the table

Instruments

- Regular laparotomy set of instruments
- Moynihan's gastric clamp (non-crushing)
- Doyen's intestinal clamp (non-crushing)
- Lane's twin gastrojejunostomy clamp

Gastrostomy

This is a surgical procedure for making an opening in the stomach for drainage or feeding.

Position of patient: Supine, same as other abdominal operations.

Instruments

- Laparotomy set of instruments
- Foley's catheter
- Gastrostomy tube
- Mosquito artery forceps both straight and curved

Gastrectomy

Gastrectomy means the removal of the stomach, but total removal is rarely indicated. Partial gastrectomy (partial removal of stomach) is done usually for cancer and recurrent bleeding of the stomach. After partial gastrectomy, remaining part is anastomosed with duodenum or jejunum.

Position of the patient: Supine on the table

Instruments

- Laparotomy set of instruments
- Moynihan's gastric clamp (non-crushing)
- Doyen's intestinal clamp (non-crushing)
- Lane's twin gastrojejunostomy clamp
- Payr's crushing gastric clamp

Intestinal Anastomosis

This surgical procedure is done to anastomose two parts of the gastrointestinal tract, either end-to-end or side-to-side. End-to-end anastomosis is done when a portion of the intestine is removed due to irrepairable injury, gangrene, malignant tumour or some other reasons. Side-to-side anastomosis is done for bypass and drainage of intestinal contents.

Position of the patient: Operation is done in the supine position on the table like other abdominal surgery.

Instruments
- Laparotomy set of instruments
- Intestinal clamps of different types

Colostomy

Colostomy is an operation, where an opening is done in the colon through the abdomen for the passage of faecal matter to excrete from the body. This procedure may be a permanent or temporary measure for the passage of stool. The colostomy wound margin is fixed to the surrounding abdominal skin. One bag is fitted on the colostomy wound for collection of stool.

Position: Supine on the table.

Instrument: General laparotomy set

Surgery for Intestinal Obstruction

Here the lumen of the small or large intestine is obstructed partially or completely for many reasons. If the obstruction is not relieved by conventional method, viability of intestine may be lost after sometimes. A segment of intestine is resected and end-to-end anastomosis is performed.

Position: Supine

Instrument: Same as gastrojejunostomy set

Colectomy

A portion or whole of the colon is removed.

Proctocolectomy

Colon and rectum are removed.

In both the surgeries, ileum is anastomosed with the remaining part of the rectum or anus.

Fistulectomy

Anal fistula is a very painful abnormal tract, connecting anal canal to the perianal skin. Fistulectomy is a surgical procedure where the fistula tract is removed.

Position: Lithotomy position of patient

Instruments
- Common general surgery instruments.
- Proctoscope

Fistulotomy

In this surgery, the fistula tract is opened and drained. This helps in healing of the tract.

Position and instruments are same as above.

Sphincterotomy

An anal fissure is a small tear in the inner lining of the anal canal. It is a very painful anal condition and mostly due to tight anal sphincter. Surgery is to remove inner layer of anal sphincter which is called sphincterotomy.

Position and instruments are as above.

Surgery for Haemorrhoids

Haemorrhoids are nothing but swollen inflamed veins around the anus or lower rectum. Patients complain of bleeding through the anus with pain. In this condition, the tissues along with the veins are ligated and excised. The sphincter is also dilated manually.

Position and instruments are as above.

Surgery for Hernia

The hernia is an area of weakness or disruption of the fibromuscular tissue of the body wall leading to protusion of viscous or a part of viscous through that opening. Inguinal hernia is the most common type of hernia.

Treatment is always surgical repair of hernia, either herniotomy or hernioplasty by using tissue or mess. It may be done by a conventional method or by laparoscopy.

Position of patient: Supine for open hernioplasty and head down for laparoscopic hernioplasty.

Surgeries for Breasts

Common surgical procedures done for various breast problems such as cancer, abscess or benign tumour are as follows:

- Lumpectomy (removal of the tumour and small surrounding normal breast tissue)
- Radical mastectomy (removal of breast, chest muscles and axillary lymph nodes)
- Modified radical mastectomy (removal of breast, nipple, skin and axillary lymph nodes)
- Breast biopsy (part of the suspicious mass is excised for histopathological examination)
- Breast abscess drainage (incision and drainage of pus from breast abscess)
- Breast lift up surgery (excess skin removed to tighten the surrounding tissue)

Position of patient: In all these procedures, the position remains supine.

Instruments: Common general surgery instruments with fine suture materials are required.

Thyroidectomy

Surgical removal of the thyroid is called thyroidectomy. It may be:
- Hemithyroidectomy (removal of one lobe and isthmus)
- Subtotal thyroidectomy (about 8 grams of tissue retain at the lower pole, rest of the part removed)
- Partial thyroidectomy (removal of the gland in front of trachea only)
- Near total thyroidectomy (removal of both side of lobe except one lower pole is preserved); or rarely
- Total thyroidectomy (removal of entire thyroid)

Thyroidectomy is done in cases of malignancy, multinodular goiter, single nodule or cyst.

Position of patient: Head end should be raised with the extension of neck.

Instruments

- General surgical instrument sets including artery forceps, tissue forceps, scalpel with blades, needle, needle holder, scissors, tissue forceps
- Joule's retractors
- Right-angled forceps
- Bulldog clamp

CHAPTER 27

Orthopaedic Surgery

Skeletal Traction

Skeletal traction is a common orthopaedic surgical procedure. In this procedure, a Steinmann pin or K-wire or any metal hook is introduced into the bone and pulled with the help of weight. The commonest site of traction is proximal tibia in adults. The other sites are distal femur, distal tibia, olecranon and skull. The purpose of traction is either temporary immobilization as first aid or to correct some deformity. For example, proximal femoral fracture is immobilized by proximal tibial traction and flexion deformity of hip is corrected by distal femoral or proximal tibial traction.

The local site is infiltrated with the local anaesthetic solution under aseptic condition and the traction pin is introduced with the help of a drill. The pin is fitted with a Bohler's stirrup and pulled with the help of a cord.

Instruments

- Syringe (10 ml) with needle
- Scalpel blade with handle
- Artery forceps
- Sponge-holding forceps
- Steinmann pin
- Hand drill with key
- Stirrup
- Nylon cord (1.5 metre)

Bone Grafting

This is a very common operation in orthopaedics where cancellous or cortical bones are collected from iliac crest or fibula or any other bone and used to promote fracture union, to fuse a joint or to fill up a gap in the bone. The most common donor site for a cancellous bone graft is iliac crest.

Position: Supine in table

Instruments

- General surgical instruments
- Periosteum elevator
- Bone levers (assorted)
- Chisel (assorted)
- Osteotome (assorted)
- Hammer (medium size)
- Gouge (assorted)
- Bone nibbler (assorted)
- Bone cutting forceps (assorted)
- Diathermy machine
- Negative suction drain

Open Reduction and Internal Fixation (ORIF)

Open reduction and internal fixation operation is mostly done for fractures of upper and lower limb bones. Aim of operation is to perform open reduction of fracture fragments followed by internal fixation of bones. By a standard exposure technique, the skin is incised, muscles are divided, and the fracture site is opened and reduced. Then the fragments are fixed by different types of suitable implants.

Instruments

- General instruments
- Periosteum elevator
- Hohmann retractors (assorted)
- Bristow
- Bone lever

- Bone-holding forceps
- Screw driver
- Chisel (assorted)
- Hammer
- Gouze (assorted)
- Bone nibbler (straight and curved)
- Bone cutting forceps (straight and curved)
- Bone cutting saw (small)
- C-Arm

- Reduction forceps (assorted)
- Volkmann's scoop

- Plate-holding forceps
- Plate bender
- Drill, drill bits, tap
- Osteotome (assorted)
- Screw assorted)
- Awl
- Bradol
- Pliar
- Wire cutting forceps

- k-wire/nail/reamer (assorted) plate/
- Heavy duty wire cutter
- Implants

FIXATION OF TROCHANTERIC FRACTURE OF FEMUR

A proximal femur fracture is a very common fracture. To fix this fracture, three common surgeries are performed, namely:

- Dynamic hip screw (DHS) fixation
- Cannulated hip screw (CHS) fixation
- Proximal femoral nail (PFN) fixation

Dynamic Hip Screw (DHS) Fixation

Trochanteric fractures are commonly treated by this procedure using DHS. Under C-arm, the fracture is reduced and fixed with a Richard screw and barrel plate.

Position of the patient: Supine in fracture table with the affected leg in traction device.

Instruments

- Instruments required for ORIF except implants
- DHS set (kept in a box for easy identification and availability)
  - DHS angle guide
  - Drill bit (assorted size)
  - Triple reamer
  - T-handle
  - Richard screw (assorted size)
  - Compression screw
  - Threaded guidewire
  - Depth gauze
  - Tissue protector
  - Tap
  - Barrel plate (3–6 hole)
- C-Arm, diathermy and sucker machine

Cannulated Hip Screw (CHS) Fixation

This procedure is done for the fracture neck of femur. Three or four cannulated screws are inserted into the neck of femur under the guidance of C-Arm.

Position of the patient: Supine in fracture table with the leg in traction

Instruments

- Instruments required for ORIF except implants
- CHS set (kept in a box for easy identification and availability)
  - CHS angle guide
  - Threaded guidewire

- Drill bit (assorted size)
- Depth gauge
- Power drill
- Cannulated tap
- Cannulated screws (assorted size)
- Cannulated screw driver
- C-Arm, diathermy and sucker machine.

Proximal Femoral Nailing (PFN)

Proximal femoral nailing is usually done for fixation of an unstable trochanteric fracture of femur. After reduction of fracture, one nail is introduced into the proximal part of femur. Under C-Arm guidance, one screw is inserted into the neck of femur with the help of a zig fitted in the proximal end of the nail percutaneously (closed method). Another screw is passed through the distal end of the nail in the same way.

Position of the patient: Supine in fracture table with leg in traction.

Instruments

- General orthopaedic instruments
- C-arm, diathermy and sucker machine
- PFN set
  - Curved and straight bone awl
  - Reaming rod
  - Guidewire-holding forceps
  - Ram guide rod
  - Tissue protector
  - Hand drill
  - Drill sleeve
  - Screw driver
  - Depth gauge
  - Medullary tube
  - Guidewire plain and also with olive point
  - Flexible reamer (assorted)
  - Ram
  - Wrench
  - Aiming trocar
  - Power drill
  - Drill bits (assorted)
  - Fixation bolt
  - PFN jig
  - Hand reamer (assorted)

Nailing of Femur and Tibia

Nailing of long bones like femur and tibia have almost same requirement for instrumentation. In this procedure, fractures of the shaft of long bones are fixed by an intramedullary nail through their proximal end.

Position of Patient

- **Femur:**
  - Commonly supine in fracture table with the affected leg in traction.
  - The lateral position with the fracture site above and a pillow in between two knees
- **Tibia:** Supine position in the plain table with radiolucent top and a firm pillow behind the knee.

Instruments

- General orthopaedic instruments
- PFN set
- Femoral or tibial or combined jig
- C-Arm, diathermy and sucker machine.

Distal Femoral Nailing (DFN)

This procedure involves the introduction of the nail through distal end of femur (through knee joint). Indication is the fracture of the distal shaft of femur.

Patient's position: Supine with the knee at 90° flexion.

Instruments: Same as that of PFN except distal femoral jig which should be added in the list.

TENSION BAND WIRING (TBW) FOR FRACTURE PATELLA

Tension band wiring is a surgical procedure where fracture fragments are aligned and fixed with K-wire and SS wire and after fixation a compressive force is created at the fracture site when the knee is flexed.

Position: Supine on the table.

Instruments

- General orthopaedic instruments
- Patella holding forceps

- K-wires of different diameter
- Stainless steel wire of different gauge.

Total or partial patellectomy: ORIF set with SS wires are necessary.

Fixation of Tibial Plateau Fracture

Different types of fracture occur in the proximal part of tibia. These are treated by ORIF mostly using side specific and fracture fragment specific plates. Requirement of instruments is the same as ORIF set along with special plates and cannulated screws.

Fixation of Fractures Around Ankle

Fractures of medial malleolus are treated either by malleolar screws or tension band wiring. Lateral malleolar fractures are fixed by distal fibular plate or small dynamic compression plate (DCP).

Position: Supine on plain table with radiolucent top.

Instruments

- ORIF set
- Distal fibular plate or Recon plate or small DCP
- C-Arm, diathermy machine and sucker machine.
- Special implants if needed.

Fixation of Fractures of Talus and Calcaneum

Same instrumentation as fractures around ankle is required. In addition, specially designed calcaneal plates are required sometimes.

Fractures of Short and Long Bones of Hands and Feet

These fractures of metatarsal, metacarpal, phalangeal bones are fixed by K-wires or mini-plate and screws according to fracture pattern.

Position: Supine on the table

Instruments

ORIF set and mini-plate screws (all instruments should be fine for such delicate surgeries).

Fixation of Clavicle Fracture

Fractures of the clavicle are usually fixed by specially designed plates, if they are not treated by closed percutaneous pinning or by conservative method.

Position: Supine on table with radiolucent top.

Instruments

- ORIF set
- Special plate for clavicle
- K-wire or TENS
- C-Arm, diathermy and suction machine.

Surgery for Proximal Humerus Fractures

For proximal humerus fracture, usually three types of surgeries are done, namely ORIF using proximal humeral plate, percutaneous K-wire fixation and shoulder arthroplasty.

Position: Supine on the table with a small sand bag behind the scapula.

Instruments

- ORIF set
- K-wires (assorted and threaded)
- Proximal humeral plate
- Arthroplasty set

Surgery for Fracture Shaft of Humerus

Plating and nailing are common surgical procedures for fracture shaft of humerus. The requirement of instruments is same as in ORIF. Only special plates and nails are added in the instrument trolley.

Fractures around Elbow

- Supracondylar fracture of humerus
- Lateral condylar fracture of humerus
- Epiphyseal injury of proximal radius
- Monteggia fracture
- Fracture radial head
- Fracture olecranon
- Intercondylar fractures of humerus
- Fracture capitellum

Fixation for the above fractures requires instruments as in ORIF set. For intercondylar fractures, specially designed lateral or medial column plates are very often asked by the surgeons. In case of comminuted radial head fracture in adult, excision or replacement is the choice.

Forearm bone fractures: ORIF set.

Distal radius fracture: ORIF set with special plates

Replacement Arthroplasty

This is one of the commonest surgical procedures in orthopaedics, where one or both components of joints are replaced by another material of similar shape and size.

When one component of the joint is replaced it is called hemiarthroplasty and when both components are replaced it is called total arthroplasty.

Hip, knee, elbow, shoulder joints are commonly replaced for different reasons. For example, in fracture neck of femur of elderly patient's femoral head is replaced by a metallic head. This is called hemiarthroplasty of hip joint.

Position: It depends on the joint and choice of the surgeon.

Instruments

- General orthopaedic instruments
- Jigs for component preparation of the joint like TKR or THR set
- Prosthesis (for example, in THR, femoral stem and head and acetabular cup available in different materials)

Spinal Fixation

Spinal fixation surgery is required in various clinical conditions of the spine-like fracture, infection, degenerative diseases, deformity and tumour.

In this surgery, two or more vertebrae are fixed by screws, rods, hooks and wires. In addition laminectomy, intervertebral disc removal, removal of tumour or correction of deformity like scoliosis and kyphosis is done, depending on the basic pathology.

Spinal fusion is required sometimes using a cage (metallic perforated container filled with bone graft) between two adjacent vertebral bodies.

Position: Most of the spinal surgeries are performed in prone position putting the patient in spinal frame. But other spinal surgeries are done either in supine or lateral position.

Instruments

- General orthopaedic set
- Spinal instrumentation set (includes all instruments required for exposure of the spine and fixation set with screws, rods and wires
- Special implants depending on the type of surgery
- C-Arm machine, sucker machine with a special metallic tube, bipolar diathermy.

Deformity Correction

Deformities correction of the upper and lower limbs are done by either by conventional method where an osteotomy is done to correct the deformity or by the Illizarov method.

Position: Supine, prone or lateral depending on the type of deformity and operation.

Instruments

- ORIF set
- Special fixation plates or nails or any other devices
- Illizarov type of external fixation set
- Limb reconstruction system (LRS) instrumentation set

Arthroscopy

Arthroscope used to visualize the internal structures of a joint. This is a machine by which a surgeon can visualize the internal structures of a joint. Common joints where it is used are knee, shoulder, hip, elbow, ankle and wrist. Arthroscope helps to diagnose and treat many joint diseases and injuries.

CHAPTER 28

Gynaecological and Obstetric Surgery

Dilatation and Curettage

This is a very common gynaecological operation where the cervix is dilated and the inner layer of uterus is scraped with sharp curette. The material is examined to detect uterine pathology including uterine cancer.

Position of patient: Lithotomy

Instruments

- Sponge-holding forceps
- Towel forceps
- Allis forceps
- Artery forceps
- Kidney dish
- Speculum (different types)
- Dilators (assorted)
- Uterine sound
- Jacob vulsellum
- Curette
- Scissors
- Thumb forceps
- Needle holder and needle

Endometrial Biopsy

A piece of the endometrium is taken from the scraped material after dilatational and curettage (as described in previous procedure) and sent for histopathological examination. This procedure is called endometrial biopsy.

Cervical Biopsy

A small part of the cervix is removed and sent for histopathological examination in this procedure.

Different Types of Biopsies

- **Punch biopsy:** Circular blade is used to take cervical tissue from multiple sites.
- **Cone biopsy:** Cone-shaped large amount of cervical tissue is collected

Position of patient: Lithotomy

Instruments

- Instruments as in D & C
- Special type of knife
- Punch forceps

Hysterectomy

This procedure involves the removal of uterus with or without ovaries, fallopian tube and cervix as per the indications of operation and underlying pathological conditions. Removal may be abdominal or vaginal. It might be laparoscope-assisted vaginal hysterectomy also.

Position of patient: Lithotomy in vaginal hysterectomy and supine in abdominal hysterectomy.

Instruments

- Common general surgical instruments as required in laparotomy
- DeBakey tissue forceps
- Mixter right angle forceps
- Deaver retractor (assorted)
- Hysterectomy forceps
- Vaginal speculum

Myomectomy

In this procedure, fibroids are removed from the uterus. Myomectomy may be abdominal open surgery or laparoscopic myomectomy.

Position of patient: Supine

Instruments

- Instruments as required in open abdominal hysterectomy
- Myoma screw
- Myoma knife
- Laparoscope with hand instruments for laparoscopic myomectomy

Colposcopy

This is a procedure by which opening of the cervix and vagina is seen more clearly and a sample of tissue is collected for examination in the laboratory.

Position: Lithotomy

Instruments

- Common general surgical instruments
- Colposcope (one device with light at the end)

Surgery for Uterine Prolapse

When pelvic floor muscles and ligaments weaken and stretch, the uterus slips down due to a lack of support. Ultimately uterus comes out of the vagina. This is called prolapsed uterus. In this condition, pelvic floor muscles are repaired. If the prolapse is severe uterus is removed. Pelvic floor repair (PFR) can be done through vagina or abdomen.

Position: Lithotomy in vaginal approach and supine in the abdominal approach.

Instruments: As required in vaginal and abdominal hysterectomy.

Caesarean Section

It is a surgical procedure in which an incision is made on the lower parts of the abdomen and uterus to deliver the newborn baby.

Position of patient: Supine

Instruments

- General laparotomy set
- Richardson retractor
- Deaver retractor
- Mayo scissors
- Umbilical scissors
- Bandage scissors
- Towel clip with ball stop
- Babcock tissue forceps
- Tissue holding forceps with triangular serrated jaws

Dilation and Evacuation

It is a process of dilation of the cervix and evacuation of the contents of uterus. This is a kind of abortion.

Position of patient: Lithotomy

Instruments

- Instruments as required in D & C set
- Suction machine with sucker tube
- Ovum forceps

Surgery for Molar Pregnancy

In molar pregnancy, there is unusual growth of placenta and converts into a fluid-filled sac and, therefore, fetus is unable to grow normally. The pregnancy is lost. It requires dilation of cervix, curettage and suction through a tube for complete removal of uterine contents.

Position: Lithotomy

Instruments: Same as dilatation and evacuation.

Tubal Ligation

This is a procedure for sterilization in which the woman's fallopian tube is clamped or blocked or sealed so that the egg from the ovary cannot reach the uterine cavity for implantation.

Position: Supine

Instruments: General surgical instruments.

Recanalization of Tube after Tubal Ligation

This procedure aims at anastomosis of both lateral and medial end of the fallopian tube. It is done under anaesthesia through usually abdominal approach. There are many other methods of recanalization of tube.

CHAPTER 29

Ophthalmic and Otorhinolaryngologic Surgery

OPHTHALMIC SURGERY

Cataract Surgery

When the lens of the eye becomes progressively opaque it causes blurry vision and affects normal activities of daily life. This clinical condition is called cataract. Treatment is the removal of lens and replacement by an artificial lens. This procedure may be:

- *Phacoemulsification* by a small incision over cornea (The lens is broken in multiple fragments and removed by suction.)
- *Extracapsular cataract extraction (ECCE)* by larger incision over the cornea (Lens is removed as single piece through larger incision.)

After removal of the lens, an artificial lens is introduced (IOL)

Position of the patient: Supine

Instruments

- Eye wire speculum
- Castro suture forceps
- McPherson STR forceps
- McPherson angle tying forceps
- Ultrashort handle forceps
- Vannas curved capsulotomy scissors
- Lens manipulating hook
- Nucleus chopper angled
- Nucleus manipulator
- Air injection cannula
- Corneal gill lightly knifes

Glaucoma Surgery

Normally, the clear fluid (aqueous humour) flows in and out of the anterior chamber and nourishes the tissues around and extra fluid is drained out of the eye. But in the certain pathological conditions, the fluid builds up but drained very slowly, which results in raised intraocular pressure. This raised pressure may damage the optic nerve and diminishes vision gradually. The aim of operations is to improve drainage of fluid and to reduce intraocular pressure.

Trabeculectomy is one operation where a small hole is created at the junction of cornea and sclera for the better outflow of aqueous humour.

Trabeculoplasty is another operation where a tiny hole is made with the laser at the filtration angle where the cornea and iris meet, for the outflow of the fluid.

Besides the above operations, small shunts and stents are inserted into the eye to increase outflow of fluid and thereby to reduce intraocular pressure.

Position of the patient: Supine

Instruments

- Common eye surgery instruments as in cataract surgery
- Trabeculectomy microhook (left and right)
- Trabeculectomy probe
- Synechiotomy glaucoma scissors
- Cleaning cannula
- Trabeculectomy probe forceps
- Spatula
- Punch Descemet's membrane
- Laser instruments for laser-assisted trabeculoplasty

Surgery for Stye and Chalazion

In the eyelid, there are oil glands. Some are opening on the inner side of the eyelid (Meibomian gland) and some on the outer side of the lid (gland of Zeis). These glands may be infected by *Staphylococcus aureus*.

Stye also called hordeolum is of two types. The infection of gland of Zeis is called hordeolum externum and hordeolum internum is infection of Meibomian gland. A chalazion is a blocked oil gland without infection.

In all these conditions, patients present a small painful lump in the eyelid with a sensation of foreign body.

Surgery

One small incision is made on the bump and contents are removed either under general or local anaesthesia.

Position of the patient: Supine

Instruments

- General eye surgery instruments
- Chalazion scoop
- Chalazion curette with serration and round type
- Meibomian gland forceps
- Chalazion clamp

Retinal Detachment Surgery

The retina is a layer of tissue at the back of the eyeball which is highly light-sensitive. Light from the exterior reaches the retina through the lens and a visual message from the retina via optic nerve goes to the brain. In pathological condition, the retina is detached from its bed and vision is lost. The surgical procedure attempts to reattach the retina to its original position.

Position of the patient: Supine

Instruments

- Common eye surgery instruments
- Cannulas
- Corneal markers
- Forceps
- Hooks and manipulators
- Retractors
- Scissors
- Speculum

Corneal Grafting/Corneal Transplant

When the cornea is damaged partially or totally it is replaced by the cornea collected from a recently dead individual with no known diseases. This is called corneal grafting or keratoplasty.

Position of the patient: Supine

Instruments

- Common eye surgery instruments
- Adjustable speculum
- Bulldog clip
- Cornea grafting scissors
- Cornea fixation ring
- Cornea fixation ring (double)
- Cornea scissors curved blade
- Bonn suturing forceps
- Colibri toothed forceps
- Curved tying forceps
- Fine curved needle holder
- Scleral support ring
- DK retractable diamond knife
- Castroviejo corneal scissors
- McPherson tying forceps

OTORHINOLARYNGOLOGIC SURGERY

Septoplasty

Deviated nasal septum (DNS) is a known clinical problem. Patients with DNS suffer from difficulty in breathing and snoring because it causes partial obstruction of airflow through the nose. The nasal septum is formed by nasal bone and cartilage. The symptoms are relieved when airflow through the nose is not obstructed. The surgical procedure of correcting DNS is called septoplasty.

Position of the patient: Supine

Instruments

- Common surgical instruments like artery forceps, Allis forceps, thumb forceps
- Speculum
- Straight and curved scissors
- Chisel
- Elevators
- Nasal forceps
- Hooks
- Knives
- Osteotomes
- Punch
- Alveolar retractors
- Rasp
- Trocar
- Suction tube

Rhinoplasty

This is a cosmetic surgery where the reshaping of the nose is done. Cuts are made within the nostrils, across the base of the nose, nasal bone and cartilage to change the shape of the nose.

Position of the patient: Supine

Instruments: Same as required for septoplasty.

Functional Endoscopic Sinus Surgery

The maxillary, ethmoid and other sinuses are cavities that produce mucous and drained outside through the nose. The sinuses may be infected which is called sinusitis. The reason is blocked drainage passage of sinuses and patients complain of stuffiness of nose, headache and thick discharge from the nose. The endoscopic surgery aims to clear the passage of the sinuses for better drainage. The surgical procedure may involve cutting of bone or removal of nasal polyp or tumour.

Position of the patient: Supine

Instruments

- Sinuscope
- Light cable and source
- Suction tube
- Suction raspatory
- Nasal speculum
- Biopsy and grasping forceps
- Nasal cutting forceps
- Antrum punch assorted
- Antrum grasping forceps and curette
- Frontal sinus punch
- Sinuscopy trocar
- Irrigation cannula
- Bipolar forceps
- Sickle knife

Surgery for Nasal Polyp

A nasal polyp is a swelling in the nasal cavity may or may not be visible from outside. It may block drainage passage of sinuses and patients may suffer from persistent nasal discharge, sinus infection and loss of the sense of smell. When drug treatment is unsuccessful, surgery is considered for removal of nasal polyp.

Position of the patient: Supine

Instruments

- Endoscope for sinus surgery
- Cannulas
- Curettes
- Nasal forceps
- Knives
- Common ENT surgical instruments
- Chisels and rasps
- Elevators
- Hooks
- Needles and needle holders

- Osteotomes
- Punches and rongeurs
- Scissors—traditional and supercut
- Suction tubes
- Probes
- Retractors
- Nasal speculums
- Trocars

Tympanoplasty

This is a surgical procedure to reconstruct the perforated tympanic membrane (eardrum) or the small bones of the middle ear. A soft tissue graft of cartilage, muscle, and fascia is collected from the ear to put on the hole of the eardrum for repair.

Position of the patient: Supine

Instruments

- Ear speculum
- Aural speculum
- Dressing forceps
- Suction cannula
- Suction adaptor
- Different retractors
- Mastoid suction cannula
- Micro-crocodile forceps
- Hand retractor
- Straight and curved needle
- Sickle knife

Mastoid Surgery

Mastoid bone located behind the ear and contains air cells that drain in the middle ear. The infection of this bone (mastoiditis) is a common clinical condition. Removal of mastoid bone (mastoidectomy) is part of the treatment for chronic mastoiditis and also for chronic suppurative otitis media. Tympano-mastoidectomy is a combined surgical procedure for repair of tympanic membrane (tympanoplasty) and opening mastoid for chronic mastoiditis.

Position of the patient: Supine

Instruments

- The instruments as mentioned for tympanoplasty
- Mastoid retractor
- Aural speculum
- Mastoid gauge
- Electric burr
- Curette and scoop
- Periosteal elevator
- Crocodile forceps
- Operating microscope
- Irrigation system
- Bipolar cautery
- Bone wax diamond spur

Stapedectomy

This is a surgical procedure to remove stapes bone and replacing the same by an artificial one. It is indicated when there are otosclerosis and loss of hearing.

Position of the patient: Supine

Instruments

- Common otolaryngologic surgery instruments as in tympanoplasty
- Raspatory
- Up cutting and down cutting knife
- Spear pointed fine needle right and left
- Roller knife
- Small hook
- Stapes hook
- Footplate rasp

Myringotomy

A small hole in the eardrum is made (myringotomy) to drain fluid from middle ear. In otitis media (ear infection), myringotomy is done to drain pus from middle ear. A drainage tube is inserted for better drainage.

Tonsillectomy

Tonsillitis is inflammation of tonsil. The children are commonly the victims of this disease. They suffer from a sore throat, difficulty in swallowing, fever, headache, and refusal to eat. Usually this condition responds to conservative treatment with antibiotics but few patients need removal of tonsils or tonsillectomy for cure.

Position of the patient: Supine

Instruments

* Common general surgery instruments
* Mouth gag
* Suction tubes
* Scissors
* Curettes
* Forceps
* Tonsil knives
* Needle holders
* Triangular punches
* Retractors
* Dissector
* Snares and wire

Parotidectomy

Parotid glands (two in number) are salivary glands situated in the upper part of the neck below the ear and encroaching the cheek. The facial nerve passes through this gland and gives branches to the muscles around. The facial nerve divides the gland into the superficial and deep part. For tumours in this region, superficial or total parotidectomy is necessary. In this surgical procedure, protection of the facial nerve is very important.

Position of the patient: Supine with head-up tilting of table and head turn to opposite site.

Instruments

* Common general surgery instruments
* A special type of parotid retractors

Thyroidectomy (See Chapter 26)

Laryngoscopy with Biopsy

Laryngeal cancer is a known clinical entity. The patient may have hoarseness of voice and pain while swallowing. In that situation, laryngoscope is inserted through oral cavity to visualize the larynx including vocal cords. If there is any growth in larynx, a part of it is taken out and sent for histopathological examination. This is called biopsy procedure.

Position of the patient: Supine

Instruments

* Laryngoscope
* Hand instruments like punch and others

Laryngeal Surgery

It includes laryngectomy and micro-laryngeal surgery. This is indicated for removal of benign or malignant tumour of larynx. The laser may be used for such cases.

CHAPTER 30

Superspeciality Surgery

UROLOGICAL SURGERY

Nephrectomy

In this procedure, the kidney is removed.

Position of the patient: Lateral on the table with kidney bridge

Instruments

- General surgical instruments
- Renal clamp

Nephrostomy

An artificial opening done between the kidney and the skin which allows urinary flow from the renal pelvis to outside (urobag)

Position of the patient: Lateral

Instruments: As required in nephrectomy.

Ureteroscopy

Bladder and lower half of ureter is visualized in this procedure. Stones in urinary bladder and ureter are removed by ureteroscopy.

Position of the patient: Lithotomy

Instruments

- General surgical instruments
- Ureteroscope with hand instruments.

Ureterolithotomy

Operation for removal of stone in ureter by open or laparoscopic surgery is called ureterolithotomy.

Position of the patient: Supine

Instruments

- General surgical instruments
- Millin's retractor
- Cystolithotomy forceps
- Nephrolithotomy forceps
- Morris kidney retractor
- Renal kidney clamp
- Laparoscope, if necessary

Ureteroscopy and Lithotripsy

Ureteroscope has one camera and light which projects an image onto the monitor. The surgeon can see the interior of the ureter and the stone. After introducing the ureteroscope, the large stones of the kidney are broken into pieces (lithotripsy) by laser and removed through the ureteroscope.

Position of the patient: Lithotomy

Instruments

- General surgical instruments
- Ureteroscope

- Ultrasonic lithotripsy
- Any other lithotripsy
- Hand instruments

Transurethral Cystolitholapaxy

A rigid tube with a camera and light at the end (cystoscope) is introduced into the bladder through the urethra to visualize its interior and bladder stone can be removed by this procedure

Position of the patient: Lithotomy

Instruments
- General surgical instrument
- Cystoscope
- Lithotripsy set

Transurethral Resection of Prostate (TURP)

In benign hyperplasia of prostate, a portion of the prostate is removed by introducing a resectoscope through the urethra. The prostate can be visualized through the resectoscope.

Position of the patient: Lithotomy

Instruments
- Common general surgical instruments
- Resectoscope set

Open Surgery for Removal of Kidney Stone

When the stone is too large in size or cannot be removed by lithotripsy, the open surgery is indicated. Usually, the operation is done in a lateral or prone position depending on the location of the stone within the kidney.

Position: Lateral, supine or prone position on the table depending on the location of the stone.

Instruments
- General surgical instruments
- Millin's retractor
- Cystolithotomy forceps
- Nephrolithotomy forceps
- Morris kidney retractor
- Renal kidney clamp

Urethroplasty

This is a type of surgery where the urethra is reconstructed. Commonly done in cases of urethral stricture.

Position: Supine

Instruments
- Turner ring retractor
- Urethral dilator set
- Mastoid retractor
- Mouth gag
- Bone nibbler
- Bone cutting forceps
- Urethroplasty gouge
- Dissecting forceps

Meatoplasty

Meatoplasty means altering the external opening of the urethra.

Position and instruments: same as urethroplasty operation.

Suprapubic Cystostomy

It is a surgical procedure by which a connection is made between the urinary bladder and the skin for drainage of urine.

Position: Supine

Instruments
- General surgical instruments
- Indwelling catheter

Circumcision

Excision of the foreskin (prepuce) of the penis at the level of the corona is done in this procedure. Another method of circumcision is application of Mogen/Gomco clamp in newborn baby below 2 months of age.

Position: Supine

Instruments
- Mosquito artery forceps (straight and curved)
- Fine thumb forceps

- Scissors (small)
- Needle holder (small)
- Fine suture materials

Orchiopexy

Undescended testis moved to the scrotal sac by orchiopexy operation.

Position of patient: Supine

Instruments: General surgical instruments.

NEUROSURGERY

Craniotomy

It is a surgical procedure where a part of the skull bone is removed to expose the brain. The bone flap removed temporarily is replaced once again to cover the brain matter at the end of the main surgical procedure. This is a basic surgery indicated in many conditions like:
- Head injury
- Brain tumour
- Arteriovenous malformation
- Cerebral aneurysm
- Brain abscess
- Biopsy from brain tissue

Position: Depending upon the site of craniotomy, the position may be supine with the raised head end, lateral or prone.

Instruments

- Common general surgery instruments
- Adson's forceps
- Suction tube
- Hemostatic forceps
- Skin retractor and hook
- Raspatory farabeue
- Bone rongeur
- Laminectomy rongeur
- Bone cutting forceps
- Vascular scissors
- Hand drill
- Hudson cranial set
- Gigli saw
- Bone lever

- Dura dissector
- Dura retractor

Brain Tumour Surgery

This surgery aims to remove the tumour of the brain at different locations. After craniotomy, the tumour is removed as planned by the surgeon.

Position: Depending upon the site of craniotomy, position may be supine with the raised head end, lateral or prone.

Instruments

- Basic instruments for craniotomy as discussed in the previous surgery.
- Micro knives
- Brain knives
- Micro raspatories
- Micro ligature instruments
- Micro nerve and vessel hooks
- Galea hooks
- Micro dissectors
- Micro curettes
- Micro elevators
- Micro needle, hooks, and spatulas
- Tumour grasping forceps
- Pituitary instruments
- Drill guide and dura protector
- Scalp clips and applying forceps

Neuroendoscopy

This is a minimally invasive surgical procedure where a telescope-like device with a video camera and eyepiece on the end is introduced through a small hole in the skull. The surgeon can reach the site of pathology and can remove the tumour or its part for histopathological examination.

Skull base tumours including pituitary tumour can be removed by endonasal endoscopic surgery. Neuroendoscope is also introduced through a small hole just above eyebrow depending on the site and shape of the tumour.

Position of the patient: Supine with head fixed from sides

Instruments

- Common general instruments
- Neuroendoscope set with hand instruments

Surgery for Traumatic Brain Injury (TBI)

When the head is injured (open or closed) the functions of the brain may be disrupted. There may be vomiting, unconsciousness, giddiness, convulsions or in serious cases even death.

Usually, there is localized haematoma in the brain and intracranial pressure increases which in turn causes more functional loss of brain.

Common surgery in such cases is the removal of haematoma after craniotomy. The exact location of the lesion can be identified by CT scan and MRI.

Position: Supine

Instruments

- Craniotomy set
- Micro dissector
- Micro dura retractor
- Micro ligature instruments

PLASTIC SURGERY

Common plastic surgeries are skin grafting, reconstruction of absent or deformed body parts (e.g. reconstruction in absent thumb). Cosmetic surgeries like, breast augmentation, breast lift, hair transplant are also not uncommon.

Skin Grafting

Skin grafting is a very common procedure in plastic surgery. The donor site is defined as the area from where the skin is taken and recipient site means where the skin is transferred. Two types of grafts are there:

- Split skin graft (only superficial layer or epidermis and a viable portion of dermis is grafted)

- Full-thickness skin graft (both epidermis and dermis are grafted) and also called flap.

In split skin grafting, the epidermis is taken from the donor site by using a special skin grafting knife (Humby's knife). The skin layer is grafted over red granulation tissue or muscles but not overexposed tendon or bone. The grafted epidermis gets nutrition from underlying tissue fluid. The thigh is the common donor site for split skin graft.

There are different types of skin flaps.

- **Pedicled flap:** Where the base is attached to the donor site through which blood reaches to the distant part of the flap.
- **Free flap:** The skin flap is detached from the donor site completely and blood vessels attached to the flap are anastomosed with the vessels at the recipient area.

Position of the patient: Supine, lateral or prone depending on the site of grafting.

Instruments

- Common general instruments
- Humby's knife
- Skin grafting blade
- Thin wooden block
- Skin spreader
- Fine suture materials.

Surgery for Cleft Lip and Cleft Palate

Cleft lip and cleft palate are congenital oral and facial malformation. There is a separation of the skin of upper lip in cleft lip. Sometimes the separation extends beyond the base of the nose and includes hard palate which is known as cleft palate.

Position of the patient: Supine

Instruments

- Mouth gag
- Round handle scalpel
- Adson forceps
- Different types of cheek retractors
- Different types of scissors
- Cleft palate hook

- Cleft palate raspatory left and right
- Mucoperiosteal retractor
- Cleft palate elevator right and left
- Measuring caliper

CARDIOTHORACIC SURGERY

Thoracotomy

This is a surgical procedure to open the thoracic cavity by any recommended approach to visualize the thoracic organs like the heart, lungs, thoracic aorta, oesophagus, anterior aspect of the spine and any other objects including foreign bodies. This is a basic surgery for performing the definitive operations of any thoracic organs. Different approaches are there to access the organs. Different approaches to open thoracic cavity:

- Median sternotomy (midline incision over sternum which is divided and most of the cardiac surgeries performed through this approach)
- Posterolateral thoracotomy
- Anterolateral thoracotomy
- Bilateral anterolateral thoracotomy combined with transverse sternotomy

Instruments

- General surgical instruments
- Thoracic forceps
- Lung tissue forceps
- Doyen costal elevator
- Rib stripers and elevators
- Farabeuf costal periosteotome
- Langenbeck periosteal elevator
- Rib shears
- Rib rongeur forceps
- Rib contractor
- Rib spreader
- For sternotomy power saw and steel, sutures are required.

Lobectomy of the Lung

The left lung has 2 lobes and right lung has 3 lobes. Lobectomy means one lobe is resected.

It is indicated in cancer, tuberculosis, and fungal infection.

Position of the patient: Lateral

Instruments

- General instruments
- Thoracotomy instruments set
- Intrathoracic artery forceps
- Different types of lung retractor
- Lung grasping forceps
- Bronchus clamp
- DeBakey multipurpose clamp

Pneumonectomy

The removal of one lung is called pneumonectomy and lobectomy means the removal of one lobe of a lung whereas a segmentectomy is wedge resection of one segment of lung. There are many conditions like cancer, infection, and injury where pneumonectomy is done.

Position of the patient: Lateral

Instruments: Same as in lobectomy.

Intercostal Drainage

This is a surgical procedure where a flexible plastic tube is inserted through the chest wall into the pleural space to remove air, pus, blood, chyle from intrathoracic space. A common indication is a hemothorax or pneumothorax after chest injury or pleural effusion in pulmonary tuberculosis

Position: Sitting at 45°

Instruments

- An intercostal catheter (different sizes)
- Spigot connector/tube adaptor—2 sizes
- Scalpel blade
- Suture material

Surgery for Congenital Heart Diseases

Common congenital heart diseases are:
- Ventricular septal defect (VSD)
- Patent ductus arteriosus (PDA)

- Atrial septal defect (ASD)
- Coarctation of aorta
- Pulmonary stenosis
- Tetralogy of Fallot

One of the treatment options in the above conditions is surgical interventions to correct the defect. Different conditions require different types of operations. But the main instrumentation is almost the same in all cases except in PDA which requires ligation only. In most of the congenital defects, open heart surgery is required using the heart-lung machine.

Position: Mostly supine

Instruments

- Thoracotomy set
- Heart-lung machine
- Instruments for cardiac surgery

Surgery for Valvular Heart Diseases

Heart has four chambers—left atrium, left ventricle, right atrium, and right ventricle; and four valves—mitral valve, tricuspid valve. pulmonary valve, and aortic valve.

These valves are open and close to control the direction of the flow of blood. In valvular diseases (congenital or acquired), the valves do not close or open properly. As a result, the heart loses functions. In such situation, the valves need repair or replacement.

- Valvoplasty (repair of valves)
- Valve replacement (to replace the damaged valve)

In most cases, sternotomy is done to reach the heart and valve surgeries are done using the heart-lung machine.

Position: Supine

Instruments

- Instruments as required surgeries for congenital anomalies of the heat
- Heart-lung machine
- Prosthetic valve

Surgery for Coronary Artery Diseases

Coronary artery disease is the narrowing of a part of the coronary artery which leads to reduced blood flow to the heart and causes chest pain. To relieve chest pain, either angioplasty or coronary artery bypass graft surgery should be done.

A piece of vein or artery is collected from the leg or wrist and grafted to the coronary artery (narrowed) so that the blood can flow bypassing the narrowed artery. The surgery can be done using a heart-lung machine or in beating heart.

Position: Supine

Instruments

- Instruments as required in valve replacement
- Heart-lung machine
- Instruments for vascular surgery

CHAPTER 31

Common Surgical Emergencies

ACUTE AIRWAY OBSTRUCTION

Airway obstruction is a real emergency. The patients present with audible stridor, suprasternal retraction, and change of voice. Common causes are:

- Inhaled foreign objects
- Diphtheria
- Ludwig's angina
- Laryngitis
- Epiglottitis
- Peritonsillar abscess
- Anaphylaxis
- Chemical burn
- Facial injury

The conservative treatment with antibiotics may not relieve the symptoms and even endotracheal intubation may be difficult because visualization may not be possible in the presence of secretion or blood in the airway. Tracheostomy is indicated in this situation.

Tracheostomy

This is a surgical procedure where a circular hole is made over the second and third tracheal ring through which a tracheostomy tube is inserted. The tube is fixed in position with the help of a soft tape to prevent accidental removal of the tube.

TENSION PNEUMOTHORAX

Tension pneumothorax is a life-threatening emergency where the air is pumped into the pleural space during each inspiration due to lung injury or a ruptured emphysematous bulla. The air cannot go back during expiration because of the one-way valve present in the visceral pleura. Progressively increasing pleural cavity air pressure compresses the lung and the patients suffer from respiratory distress, chest pain with tachypnoea, tachycardia and diminished or absent breath sound.

In this situation, one wide bore needle is introduced at second intercostal space in midclavicular line to reduce intrathoracic tension. Subsequently, the intercostal drain is placed with slow suction.

Intercostal Drain

This procedure may be required both in the pre-hospital or hospital environment as a life-saving measure.

Position: Sitting or propped up

Instruments

- Wide bore needle
- Sterile gloves
- Instruments for intercostal drainage

CARDIAC TAMPONADE

Sudden accumulation of fluid or blood in pericardial space causes compression of cardiac chambers. This is called cardiac tamponade.

The common causes of intrapericardial pressure are injury or infective lesions of peri cardium. The patients suffer from hypotension with raised jugular venous pressure.

Treatment in this emergency is pericardial tap or pericardiocentesis under US guidance. Definitive treatment is pericardiotomy or pericardiectomy.

Position: Supine

Instruments

- Thoracotomy instruments set
- Wide bore needle
- US machine

Acute appendicitis: Chapter 26

Intestinal obstruction: Chapter 26

GASTROINTESTINAL PERFORATION

Perforation of the gastrointestinal tract occurs commonly due to ulcer but may be enteric or traumatic in origin. The intestinal contents come out and contaminate the peritoneal cavity. That leads to peritonitis. The patients present with acute pain and distension of abdomen with varying degrees of toxic features in late cases. The common site of perforation is duodenum.

The surgical treatment in this situation includes peritoneal toileting and repair of perforation by suturing the hole along with omental patch cover, if necessary.

ACUTE MESENTERIC ISCHAEMIA

This is a condition where the blood flow of the intestinal wall is suddenly interrupted due to embolism or thrombosis. Due to ischaemia, gangrenous changes may occur in the intestinal wall leading to peritonitis.

Immediate diagnosis is difficult but later patients present with acute pain abdomen and varying degrees of toxicity. Treatment depends on the stage of the disease.

ACUTE RETENTION OF URINE

Acute retention of urine is a common emergency condition when a patient cannot micturate even urinary bladder is full. This is a great discomfort to the patient and the cause is either obstruction in the urinary tract or weakness of the muscles of the bladder.

Treatment is immediate relief by bladder drainage with the help of simple rubber catheter (one time). Foley's catheter (for longer period) catheterization is indicated for long-term relief. Curative treatment for retention of urine is the removal of the cause, which is as follows:

- Urethral dilatation (urethral stricture)
- Resection of prostate (benign hypertrophy of the prostate)
- Removal of tumour
- Removal of stones in the passage
- Suprapubic cystostomy

Position: Supine or lithotomy depending on the procedure.

Instruments

- Instruments as required in suprapubic cystostomy
- Urethral dilators
- TURP set (Chapter 41; page 186)
- Ureteroscope
- Cystoscope

TESTICULAR TORSION

Boys between 12 and 18 years of age are usually the victims of testicular torsion. The testis rotates inside the scrotum with the spermatic cord which contains the testicular artery. Twisting causes reduced blood flow to the testis and patients feel severe pain in the scrotum. If it persists, testis suffers from ischaemia and cannot be saved. This is a real emergency. Surgical treatment involves de-torsion and fixation of the testis, if detected early but the removal of testis may be necessary in late cases.

Position of the patient: Supine

Instruments: General surgical fine instruments.

PARAPHIMOSIS

When the foreskin of the penis is retracted behind the corona of the glans and remains there as a constricting ring, impairment of distal venous and lymphatic drainage with the reduced arterial flow to the glans occurs.

This leads to swelling of the glans and foreskin with difficulty in urination. This is called paraphimosis. Phimosis, on the other hand, is a situation where the foreskin cannot be retracted to expose the glans. Paraphimosis is one of the urological emergencies. The emergency treatment protocol includes:

- Manual compression of the glans to reduce the oedema.
- Application of ice-cold water locally.
- The foreskin is relocated to its normal anatomical position.
- If it fails a small incision is made on the foreskin.

Position: Supine

Instruments: General fine surgical instruments.

BLEEDING ECTOPIC PREGNANCY

When the fertilized ovum grows outside the uterus (mostly in the fallopian tube) it is called ectopic pregnancy. This ectopic pregnancy becomes complicated with the rupture of the fallopian tube, which is an obstetric emergency. Treatment is the removal of the fallopian tube (salpingectomy).

Position: Supine

Instruments: Same as laparotomy set.

RETAINED PLACENTA WITH BLEEDING

Retained placenta is a condition when the placenta is not delivered on its own within 30 minutes of the baby's birth. The reason may be failed or incomplete separation from the uterus or the separated placenta is retained in the uterine cavity.

This may cause postpartum haemorrhage. Retained placenta is complicated with infection and haemorrhage. The patient usually presents with pain and foul-smelling vaginal discharge with large pieces of tissues. Vaginal bleeding and sepsis can be life-threatening. Management aims to prevent infection and to remove the placenta. Drugs like oxytocin, ergometrine are usually used. If conservative treatment fails, manual removal by controlled cord traction or curettage is done. Rarely hysterectomy is required for uncontrolled bleeding.

Position of the patient: Supine

Instruments

- General instruments for D & E set.
- Instruments as required for a hysterectomy to keep ready, if necessary.

Emergency Caesarean Section
(Chapter 28)

Emergency caesarean section is commonly indicated in fetal distress and antepartum haemorrhage or both. It is an obstetrical emergency.

ACUTE SUBDURAL HAEMATOMA

Acute subdural haematomas (SDHs) are the result of head injury which might be fatal sometimes. Bleeding occurs from the torn surface vessels of the brain and the blood is collected under the dura mater. The large haematomas create pressure effects on the brain with altered consciousness levels having low Glasgow Coma Scale. The SDHs are best detected by CT scan and if it is 1 cm in thickest point, drainage is indicated. Drainage and decompression are done by standard craniotomy surgery on the site of haematoma detected by CT scan.

RUPTURED AORTIC ANEURYSM

The aneurysm is localized abnormal swelling in the wall of an artery. The rupture of aortic aneurysm is common in abdominal aorta in persons above 50 years of age. The patients with ruptured abdominal aortic aneurysm (AAA) have pain abdomen, hypotension, and a pulsatile abdominal mass. This is a real surgical emergency as the patients are in severe hypovolemic shock due to the rupture of a major vessel's aneurysm.

After resuscitation, ultrasound examination is done to confirm the diagnosis. There are two methods of repair—endovascular aneurysm repair (EVAR) and open repair. EVAR interventional radiology service should be available in operation theatre. Open repair is done in an operation theatre where facilities of vascular surgery are available. The interventional radiologist and vascular surgeon with the help of anaesthesiologist perform this job.

Position: Supine

Instruments

- Cannulas
- Aneurysm clips and appliers
- Vascular clamps
- Dilators
- Elevators
- Forceps
- Hooks
- Needle holders and needles
- Retractors

INTERNAL BLEEDING

Internal bleeding is not visible and it is of great concern when the amount of extravasated blood causes symptoms in the body. The cause of the bleeding may be traumatic or non-traumatic.

- **Traumatic**
  a. A blunt injury where no external injury is found (rupture of the spleen in sports injury).
  b. Penetrating injury where the external injury is found but the bleeding point may not be visible. Common example is gun-shot injury to the abdomen with bleeding from mesenteric vessels.

- **Non-traumatic:** It may be due to some medical, congenital or neoplastic reasons like bleeding from gastric ulcer or rupture of arteriovenous malformation in the brain.

Symptoms and signs of internal bleeding depend on its locations and severity. It may be slight dizziness to unconsciousness with tachycardia and hypotension.

Subdural haematomas and haemopneumothorax are common examples of internal bleeding. The goal of treatment is to stop bleeding.

After resuscitation, investigations like X-ray, CT scan, MRI, ultrasonogram are suggested to locate the site and amount of bleeding. The bleeding sites are exposed (craniotomy, thoracotomy, laparotomy) and the bleeding vessels are ligated. Large vessels need repair like popliteal or brachial arteries.

Position: Supine or prone depending on the locations.

Instruments: Craniotomy, thoracotomy, laparotomy instrument set as necessary.

Section V
Anaesthesia and Common Perioperative Complications

CHAPTER 32

Classifications of Anaesthesia

The word anaesthesia is coined from two Greek words, *"an"* means without and *"aesthesia"* means sensation. Therefore, anaesthesia is a branch of modern medicine deals with the administration of medications that block the feeling of pain and other sensations.

Anaesthesia is a state of controlled, temporary loss of sensation or awareness that is induced to conduct various surgical or invasive procedures without any pain or discomfort. It includes analgesia (relief from pain), paralysis (muscular relaxation), amnesia (loss of memory) and unconsciousness.

CLASSIFICATION

All the types of anaesthesia are administered to keep patients comfortable and pain-free during surgery, invasive procedures or painful diagnostic test. Different types of anaesthesia are classified under four categories:

- General anaesthesia
- Monitored sedation
- Regional anaesthesia
- Local anaesthesia

General Anaesthesia

To conduct any surgical procedure, the patient is made unaware or unresponsive to the painful stimuli by administering general anaesthetic agents. General anaesthesia is used for major operations such as laparotomy, thoracotomy, etc. and causes the patient to lose consciousness.

Monitored Sedation

Sedation is often used for minimally invasive procedures like endoscopies to relieve discomfort associated with such procedures. The level of sedation ranges from minimal to deep sedation.

Regional Anaesthesia

It is a type of anaesthesia where pain associated with surgery is relieved by producing a reversible loss of sensation of a part of the body. A local anaesthetic agent is deposited near a peripheral nerve or central neuraxis and cause temporary loss of transmission of sensation. Regional anaesthesia includes:

- Peripheral nerve blocks
- Plexus blocks
- Central neuraxial blocks

Peripheral Nerve Blocks

Local anaesthetic agent deposited near peripheral nerves and blocks the transmission of sensation. Common nerve blocks are as follows.

- Retrobulbar nerve block (nerve block for ophthalmic surgery)
- Ulnar and radial nerves block
- Intercostal nerve block
- Nerve blocks on lower extremity
  - Femoral nerve block
  - Sciatic nerve block
  - Obturator nerve block
  - Lateral cutaneous femoral nerve block
  - Blocks of five nerves to achieve ankle block
    - Deep peroneal nerve
    - Superficial peroneal nerve
    - Saphenous nerve
    - Posterior tibial nerve
    - Sural nerve

Plexus Blocks

- **Cervical plexus block:** Blocks C1–C4 spinal nerve.
  - *Indications:*
    - Operations in the neck region
    - Cervical lymph node biopsy
    - Carotid endarterectomy
    - Thyroid surgery
- **Brachial plexus block:** Blocks C4–T2 spinal nerve roots
  - *Indications:* Operations of the upper extremity
- **Lumbar plexus block:** Blocks L1–L4 spinal nerve roots
  - *Indications:* May be used along with sciatic nerve block for lower limb surgery
    - Operations for fracture neck femur
    - Operations for fracture shaft femur
    - Knee operations
    - Operations on the anterior part of the thigh

Central Neuraxial Block

It is a type of regional anaesthesia that involves the injection of anaesthetic medication in the fatty tissue that surrounds the nerve roots as they pierce and pass through epidural space (known as epidural and caudal) or into the cerebrospinal fluid which surrounds the spinal cord (known as the subarachnoid or spinal block)

- **Subarachnoid block (spinal anaesthesia):** Local anaesthetic agent is deposited at subarachnoid space and blocks nerves passing through the cerebrospinal fluid.
  - *Saddle block:* Produces sensory block of lower lumbar and sacral segments.
  - *Low spinal:* Blocks up to umbilical (T10) level
  - *Mid spinal:* Blocks up to costal margin (T6) level
  - *High spinal:* Blocks up to nipple line (T4) level
- **Epidural anaesthesia:** Local anaesthetic agent is deposited in epidural space and blocks the nerve passes through epidural space.
  - Cervical epidural
  - Thoracic epidural
  - Lumbar epidural
  - Caudal epidural

Local Anaesthesia

Local anaesthesia is defined as a loss of sensation in a circumscribed area of the body caused by a depression of excitation in nerve ending or inhibition of the conduction process in the peripheral nerves. It does not cause loss of consciousness. Local anaesthesia may be of following types:

- Infiltration anaesthesia
- Field block
- Surface anaesthesia

Infiltration Anaesthesia

A local anaesthetic agent is injected into the area which is to be incised in a circular manner.

Infiltration anaesthesia may be used to excised small cyst, tumour, etc.

Field Block

Zone of anaesthesia is created around the operative field by injecting local anaesthetic agent. Example: Anaesthesia for excision of breast mass.

Topical or Surface Anaesthesia

Local anaesthetic agents are administered in the form of spray, ointment, cream or lotion. They are used to anaesthetize the surface of the skin or mucous membrane.

- Surface anaesthesia is used in bladder catheterization, cystoscopy, etc.

- EMLA cream (eutectic mixture of local anaesthetic agents, i.e. lignocaine and prilocaine) is commonly used to produce surface anaesthesia.
- **Types of topical anaesthesia:**
  - Spray → refrigeration (used for boils, abscess drainage, etc.)
  - Ointment → pain relief in case of insect bites
  - Instillation → anaesthesia for urethral meatus
  - Direct contact with local anaesthetics → use of cotton pledget soaked in local anaesthetic agents for anaesthesia of nasal mucosa, etc.

CHAPTER 33

General Anaesthesia

General anaesthesia is a medically induced reversible state of unconsciousness with the inability to feel and respond to surgical or any other painful stimulus. In modern anaesthesia practice, this includes the triad of unconsciousness, analgesia and muscular relaxation.

General anaesthetics are the drugs which produce a reversible loss of all modalities of sensation and consciousness or simply drugs that bring about a reversible loss of consciousness.

STAGES OF ANAESTHESIA

Classical stages of anaesthesia are rarely seen in modern anaesthesia practice due to the introduction of potent intravenous and inhalational inducing agents. Stages of anaesthesia were described by AE Guedel in 1937, which was observed in unpremedicated patient induced by diethyl ether.

Stage 1: Stage of Analgesia

- Normal reflexes are maintained until the loss of consciousness.
- Abolition of the eyelash reflex at the end of stage 1.

Stage 2: Stage of Excitement

- Excitement

- Irregular breathing
- Struggling and resisting
- Regurgitation, coughing and laryngeal spasm
- Dilatation of pupil

Stage 3: Stage of Surgical Anaesthesia

Plane I

- Eyeball centrally placed
- Swallowing reflex depressed
- Loss of conjunctival reflex, pupil normal or small
- Increased lacrimation

Plane II

- Regular deep breathing
- Loss of corneal reflexes
- Beginning of pupillary dilatation
- Beginning of intercostal muscle paralysis

Plane III

- Shallow breathing
- Complete intercostal muscle paralysis
- Suppression of laryngeal reflex

Plane IV

- Diaphragmatic paralysis
- Depressed cranial reflex

Stage 4: Stage of Overdose

- Pupil fully dilated
- Apnoea

These classical stages of anaesthesia are not seen in modern anaesthesia practice. However, ocular movement, lacrimation and neuroendocrinal response are common during a lighter plane of anaesthesia.

General anaesthesia has the following basic components:

- Loss of modalities of sensations
- Sleep and amnesia
- Immobility or muscle relaxation
- Abolition of reflexes—somatic and autonomic

The optimal combination of anaesthetic drugs is administered by anaesthesiologist to achieve triads of unconsciousness, analgesia and muscle relaxation.

OBJECTIVES OF GENERAL ANAESTHESIA

- Unconsciousness
- Amnesia
- Analgesia
- Oxygenation
- Ventilation
- Homeostasis
- Airway management
- Reflex suppression
- Muscular relaxation
- Monitoring

STEPS OF GENERAL ANAESTHESIA

Preinduction Period

- **Intravenous cannulation:** On arrival in the operation theatre, the patient is transferred on the operation table and intravenous cannulation is performed. Intravenous infusion is started and continued throughout the surgical procedure with crystalloids, colloids and blood, if indicated.

- The intravenous channel is used to administer different anaesthetic agents during the perioperative period.
- **Monitoring:** Monitors are attached to the patient before induction of anaesthesia and baseline parameters are recorded. Monitoring is done throughout the surgical procedure. Type of monitoring depends upon the type of surgery, type of anaesthesia and physical status of the patient. Minimum monitoring during surgery may be as follows:
  - Pulse and blood pressure monitoring
  - Continuous electrocardiography (ECG)
  - Continuous pulse oximetry (SpO_2)
  - Capnography to measure end-tidal carbon dioxide
  - Monitoring of core and surface temperature
  - Respiratory gas analyser
  - Alarm systems such as low-pressure alarm, oxygen alarm and circuit disconnect alarm

Induction of Anaesthesia

This is the period which starts from the beginning of the administration of anaesthesia to achievement of the surgical plane of anaesthesia.

General anaesthesia is induced either by intravenous or inhalational anaesthetic agents. Common intravenous anaesthetic agents are thiopentone sodium, propofol, etomidate and ketamine. Induction is usually very smooth and the excitatory phase does not occur because induction is very fast and takes place within one arm brain circulation time. Sevoflurane is the most preferred inducing agent among the inhalation anaesthetic group.

Steps of Induction

- Preoxygenation, to fill the lungs with oxygen and create oxygen reserve to cope up apnoea during airway management. The inspired and end-tidal oxygen difference is the best monitor of the adequacy of preoxygenation or denitrogenation.

- Intravenous administration of analgesics preferably opioids to provide analgesia during the intraoperative period.
- Induction with inducing dose of intravenous or inhalational anaesthetic agents.
- **Management of clear airway:** Supraglottic airway devices may be used when muscle paralysis is not required and minimal risk of regurgitation. If endotracheal intubation is indicated, the correct placement of the tube must be confirmed clinically as well as by capnography. Supraglottic device or endotracheal tube must be fixed with tape or adhesive plaster to prevent displacement.
- Intravenous administration of muscle relaxant is usually indicated to facilitate laryngoscopy and intubation.

Maintenance of Anaesthesia

After induction, the surgical plane of anaesthesia is maintained throughout the operative period. Maintenance of anaesthesia is usually done with an inhalational anaesthetic agent in either air/oxygen or nitrous oxide/oxygen mixture. Other option may be a combination of intravenous agents such as propofol and short-acting opioids. A muscle relaxant is supplemented at regular intervals according to clinical and/or nerve stimulator response. The multimodal approach usually provides optimal pain relief in the postoperative period.

According to physical status and type of surgical procedures, anaesthesiologists may prefer to keep the patient on spontaneous ventilation or controlled ventilation. Adequacy of ventilation must be assessed during the perioperative period.

After induction of anaesthesia, the job of an anaesthesiologist is:

- To maintain a surgical plane of anaesthesia
- To monitor vital parameters and take appropriate action, if there is any warning sign

- To assess fluid deficits and appropriate replacement by intravenous fluids
- Prediction and prevention of complications
- Detection and management of intraoperative complications.

Depth of anaesthesia is assessed by clinical parameters such as pulse, blood pressure, lacrimation, sweating, body movement and by monitor, bispectral monitor.

Recovery of Anaesthesia

At the end of surgical procedure, administration of the anaesthetic agent is stopped for recovery from anaesthesia.

Steps of Recovery of Anaesthesia

- Turn off all the anaesthetic agents (intravenous and/or inhalational anaesthetic agents)
- Assess the degree of neuromuscular blockade by nerve stimulator and reverse the residual effect by administering anticholinesterase preceded by atropine or glycopyrronium to counteract muscarinic like effects.
- Return of spontaneous ventilation with adequate ventilation and oxygenation.
- The suction of pharynx and oral cavity to clear upper airway.
- Extubation and assessment for unobstructed upper airway.
- Assess the patient for recovery and analyze the patient response to verbal command.
- Monitor vital parameters of the patient and assess for haemodynamic stability.
- After recovery, patients are shifted to post-anaesthetic care unit for further management under closed observation and monitoring.

Emergence is the return of physiological functions of the central nervous system after cessation of general anaesthetics. There may be temporary neurologic phenomenon such as emergence delirium, impaired comprehensive speech and/or focal impairment of sensory or motor functions.

Inadequate ventilation and hypoxaemia are common during the immediate postoperative period. Cardiovascular events such as increased blood pressure, pulse rate and dysrhythmias are also observed in the immediate postoperative period.

DUTIES OF OPERATION THEATRE TECHNOLOGIST

- Check anaesthesia machine, vapourizers and anaesthesia breathing system.
- Check difficult airway cart and ensure all instruments are in order.
- Check the functional status of the suction machine. Ensure the availability of different sizes of the suction catheter.
- Check the functional status of all monitors. After transfer of the patient to the operation table, attach all monitors and record baseline parameters.
- Continuous monitoring and recording of the vital parameters during the operative procedure.
- Check emergency drug tray and ensure the availability of all emergency drugs.
- Establish intravenous channel and initiate fluid therapy.
- Assist anaesthesiologist during laryngoscopy and endotracheal intubation.
- Draw anaesthetic drugs and label the syringe, preferably with colour coding.
- Assist anaesthesiologist by recording vital parameters at regular intervals.
- Assist anaesthesiologist during reversal of anaesthesia, extubation, recovery and transfer of the patient to post-anaesthesia care unit.

Regional Anaesthesia

A specific part of the body is made insensitive to painful stimuli by blocking the conduction of nerves. It can be a peripheral nerve block or central neuraxial block.

PERIPHERAL NERVE BLOCK

Peripheral nerves may be blocked at any points along their path. To achieve sensory and motor blockade, local anaesthetic agents are deposited as close to the nerve as possible without touching the nerve itself. The success of nerve blocks depends upon the accurate location of nerve and deposition of local anaesthetic agents at a proper plane.

The nerve can be located by a nerve stimulator or portable ultrasound device.

Nerve Stimulator (Fig. 34.1)

Peripheral nerve stimulators transmit a small electric current to the tip of the needle to stimulate neural structure close to it and contract muscles supplied by such nerve. Nerve stimulator helps to locate peripheral nerve without damaging it.

- Nerve stimulator helps to deposit local anaesthetic agent accurately close to the targeted nerve.
- It consists of two leads. The positive lead is connected to an ECG skin electrode and the negative lead is attached to locating needle.

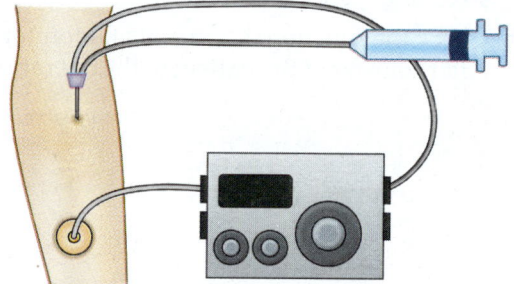

Fig. 34.1: Peripheral nerve stimulator

- A constant current of 0.25–0.5 mA is used to stimulate the targeted nerve and there is a contraction of muscles supplied by the nerve.
- Duration of each stimulus is 1–2 Hz. Each stimulus causes painless muscle contraction.
- The nerve stimulator is battery operated.
- The nerve stimulator is connected to nerve block needle.

Nerve Block Needles

- They are made of steel and have Luer-lock attachment.
- The bevel of the needle is short and blunt which increases the resistance, improves feedback feeling and minimizes the chance of nerve trauma.

- There are two types of needles: (a) Insulated needle and (b) non-insulated needle.
- **Insulated needles:** Except the tip of the needle, they are coated with 'Teflon'. Therefore, current passes only through the tip.
- **Non-insulated needles:** Current passes through the tip as well as the shaft of the needle. Therefore, a higher range of current is necessary to stimulate nerve fibres.
- Needles have a transparent hub for early detection of intravascular placement of the tip of the needle.
- The needle is connected to a nerve stimulator to locate the nerve targeted for the block.
- Side port of the needle is used to connect with a syringe and inject local anaesthetic agent.
- Size of the needle is 22 gauges and length varies according to the depth of the nerve or plexus.
- **Length of needles:**
  - Interscalene block—25–50 mm
  - Axillary block—25–50 mm
  - Femoral nerve block—50 mm
  - Psoas compartment block—75–125 mm
  - Sciatic nerve block—75–150 mm

Ultrasound Machine

- The ultrasound machine is used for visualization of the target nerve, position of the needle and the deposition of local anaesthetics around the nerve.
- Ultrasound is a longitudinal high-frequency sound wave (above the human audible range). Ultrasound is created by converting electrical energy into mechanical vibration by the piezoelectric effect (PE). An image is formed when the ultrasound wave is transmitted into the body, reflected from tissue and returned to the transducer.
- Higher frequencies (10–14 MHz) give higher resolution with low tissue penetration.

They are used for superficial plexus block. Lower frequencies (4–7 MHz) are used for deeper penetration to visualize deeper structures but the resolution is not optimum.

- In the transverse plane, peripheral nerve appears as a round or oval structure consisting of hypoechoic bubbles surrounded by hyperechoic elements. In the longitudinal plane, nerves look like hypoechoic parallel bands, bordered by hyperechoic striations.

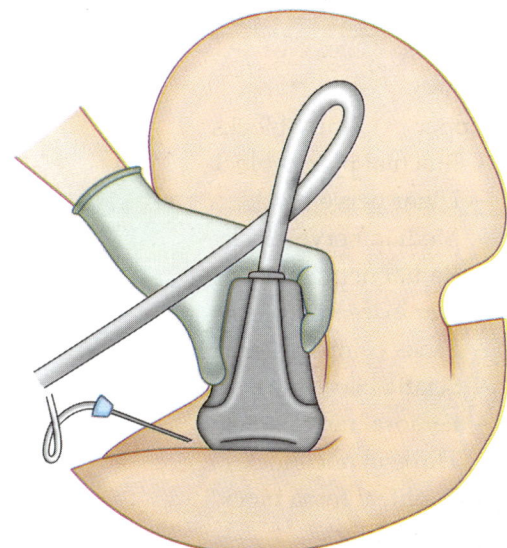

Fig. 34.2: USG-guided nerve block

- Position of the tip of the needle can be detected by an ultrasound machine. Injection of local anaesthetic agent and its spread can also be observed by this machine (Fig. 34.2).

Types of Equipment for Peripheral Nerve Blocks

- Equipment for the location of peripheral nerves: Ultrasound machine and/or nerve stimulators.
- Nerve block needles for single-shot peripheral nerve block.
- Tuohy needle with a catheter for continuous peripheral nerve blocks.

- The antiseptic solution, sterile gauze pieces, gloves and sponge holding forceps for preparing sterile zone at the site of block.
- Commonly used local anaesthetic agents for peripheral nerve block:

Local anaesthetics	The concentration of local anaesthetics
Lignocaine	1 to 2%
Bupivacaine	0.25 to 0.5%
Levobupivacaine	0.25 to 0.5%
Ropivacaine	0.2 to 0.5%

Commonly used Nerve Blocks

- Upper extremity blocks
  - Brachial plexus block
  - Ulnar nerve block
  - Median nerve block
  - Radial nerve block
- Lower extremity blocks
  - Psoas compartment block
  - Sciatic nerve block
  - Femoral nerve block
  - Three in one block
  - Popliteal fossa block
  - Ankle block
- Blocks of head and neck
  - Trigeminal nerve block
  - Cervical plexus block
  - Blocks for upper airway anaesthesia
  - Stellate ganglion block
  - Retrobulbar and peribulbar blocks
- Blocks for thorax and abdomen
  - Intercostal nerve block
  - Coeliac plexus block
  - Paravertebral block
  - Ilioinguinal and iliohypogastric block
  - Penile block

CENTRAL NEURAXIAL BLOCK

Central neuraxial block is the method to interrupt neuronal transmission at the level of nerve roots as they emerge from the spinal cord.

Central neuraxial blockade is obtained by:

- Intradural or subarachnoid anaesthesia (spinal anaesthesia)
- Extradural anaesthesia
- Combined intradural-extradural anaesthesia (CSE or combined spinal-epidural anaesthesia)
- Continuous intradural anaesthesia

Subarachnoid Anaesthesia

- In subarachnoid block, the local anaesthetic agent is deposited in subarachnoid space after dural puncture. The drug is diffused into the cerebrospinal fluid.
- Commonly it is known as spinal anaesthesia.
- Single-shot spinal anaesthesia is simple to administer with rapid onset and recovery of sensory and motor block.

Extradural Anaesthesia

- A local anaesthetic agent is deposited in the epidural space.
- Epidural space is a potential space situated between ligamentum flavum and dura mater. It is bounded cranially by foramen magnum and caudally by sacrococcygeal ligament overlying sacral hiatus. Anteriorly and posteriorly, epidural space is bounded by posterior longitudinal ligament and ligamentum flavum plus vertebral laminae, respectively. It contains nerve roots, blood vessels and epidural fat.
- Epidural anaesthesia can be done in any vertebral interspace irrespective of the level of termination of the spinal cord.

Combined Intradural and Extradural Anaesthesia

- It is commonly known as combined spinal-epidural (CSE) anaesthesia.
- In this technique, a spinal block is given by single-shot technique and an epidural catheter is placed in epidural space to deposit local anaesthetic agent and continue block as long as it is indicated.
- It combines the advantage of quick onset effect of spinal anaesthesia and prolonged duration of actions through continuous infusion of local anaesthetics by the epidural catheter.

Continuous Intradural Anaesthesia

- Microcatheter is introduced in subarachnoid space to deposit local anaesthetic agents continuously.
- Continuous intradural anaesthesia is used when epidural anaesthesia is either difficult or contraindicated.

Preparation for Central Neuraxial Block

- Preoperative assessment, preparation and consent for operation and anaesthesia.
- Obtain venous access and start intravenous infusion.
- Attach monitors and record baseline parameters (pulse, blood pressure, ECG, oxygen saturation, etc.).
- Check anaesthesia machine and resuscitative trolley.
- Check emergency drugs including anaesthetic agents.
- Check the operating table for change in height and tilt.
- Check the functional status of a defibrillator.

POSITION OF THE PATIENT

Sitting Position

- Anatomical midline is easier to identify in sitting position.
- The sitting position is especially preferred in obese patients.
- The patient is placed across the table with feet resting comfortably on a stool.
- The spine should be flexed with the chin is pressed onto the sternum (Fig. 34.3).
- A pillow on the knees gives support to the arms.
- Flexion of the spine maximizes the 'target area' between the adjacent spinous process and brings the spine closer to the skin surface.

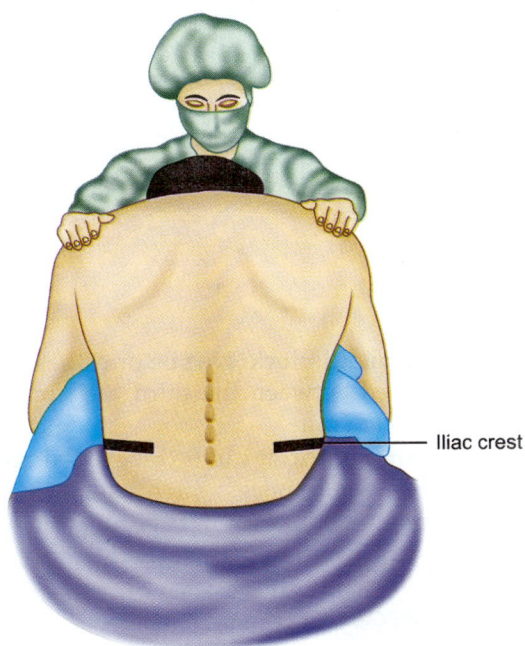

— Iliac crest

Fig. 34.3: Sitting position for neuraxial block

Lateral Position

- The patient is placed on a lateral position with his or her back parallel to the edge of the table. The lower limb is flexed at hip and knee joints in such a way that it comes nearer to the abdomen. Head is also flexed.
- An assistant helps the patient to assume and hold this position (Fig. 34.4).

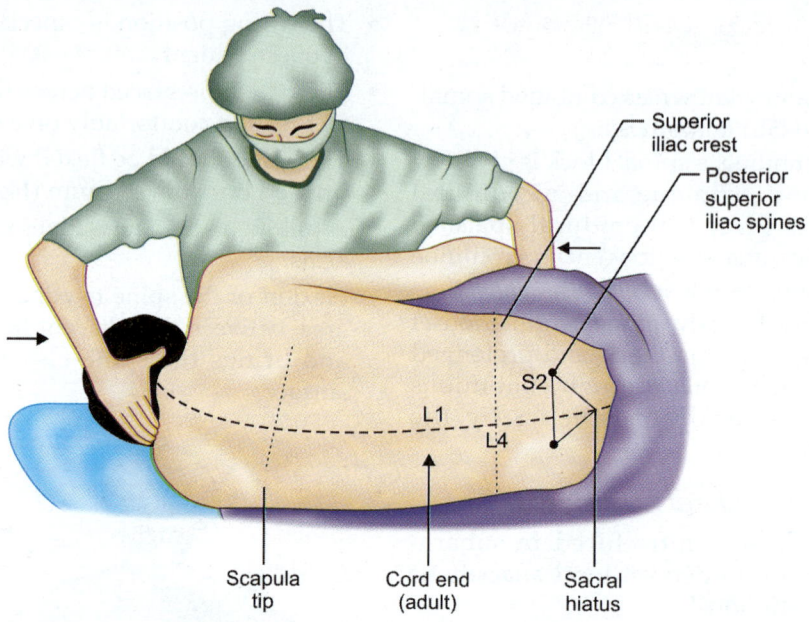

Fig. 34.4: Lateral position for neuraxial block

Site of Insertion of a Needle for Central Neuraxial Block

- **Subarachnoid block:** Needle or catheter is introduced between the third and fourth lumbar vertebrae.
- **Extradural block:** It can be blocked at any vertebral interspaces, such as cervical, thoracic, lumbar or caudal epidural block.

Needles for Central Neuraxial Block

Spinal Needles

- Spinal needles are used to deposit local anaesthetics and opioids into subarachnoid space.
- Length of needles varies from 5 to 15 cm.
- The stylet is used to prevent occlusion of needle lumen by a core of tissue. The stylet is withdrawn once the tip of the needle is in the subarachnoid space.
- Size of the needles varies from 18 to 29 G.
- Two types of spinal needles are available, (a) cutting traumatic bevelled needle (Yale or Quincke needles) and (b) non-cutting atraumatic pencil-point needles (Whitacre and Sprotte needles).
- Spinal microcatheter is used for continuous subarachnoid block.

Epidural Needles (Tuohy Needle)

- Tuohy needle is usually 10 cm in length and 16 to 18 G in diameter.
- Needle consists of stylet which prevents occlusion of lumen by a core of tissue.
- The bevel of the needle is curved at 20°C (Huber point) and the edge of the needle is blunt.
- The shaft of a needle is marked at intervals of 1 cm.
- The epidural catheter is usually 90 cm long. The proximal end is connected with a Luer lock and filter.
- The distal end is marked at 5 cm intervals with additional 1 cm markings between 5 and 15 cm.

Commonly used Drugs for Central Neuraxial Block

Subarachnoid Block

Local anaesthetics (%)	Dose		Duration of block
	Mid-spinal block (T10)	**High spinal block (T4)**	
Bupivacaine (0.5%)	10–15 mg	12–20 mg	130–230 min
Levobupivacaine (0.5%)	10–15 mg	12–20 mg	130–230 min
Ropivacaine (0.5–0.75%)	12–18 mg	18–25 mg	80–210 min
Lignocaine (2.0%)	40–80 mg	80–100 mg	60–120 min

Epidural Block

Local anaesthetics	Concentration (%)	Onset (min)	Duration (min)
Bupivacaine	0.5 (for analgesia 0.25–0.125)	20	165–225
Levobupivacaine	0.5	15–20	150–225
Ropivacaine	0.75	15–20	140–180
Lignocaine	2.0	15	45–60

Instruments for Central Neuraxial Block

- The sterile tray contains:
  - Spinal needle or Tuohy needle
  - Bowl with an antiseptic solution
  - Gloves
  - Sterile gauge piece
  - Sponge holding forceps
- The local anaesthetic agent with or without adjuvants

CHAPTER 35

Pharmacology and Anaesthesia

Anaesthesia is rarely achieved by a single drug. A combination of drugs is used to achieve the desired level of hypnosis, analgesia and muscle relaxants. Various dosages of hypnotics, analgesics with or without muscle relaxants are administered and achieve targeted depth of anaesthesia. Commonly used pharmacological agents are as follows.

- Inhalational anaesthetic agents
- Intravenous anaesthetic agents
- Analgesic agents
- Neuromuscular blocking agents
- Anaesthetic adjuvants
- Local anaesthetic agents (for regional anaesthesia)

INHALATIONAL ANAESTHETIC AGENTS

Inhalational anaesthetic agents are chemical compounds produce general anaesthesia. Commonly used inhalational anaesthetic agents include inorganic gas nitrous oxide and the volatile liquids isoflurane, desflurane, sevoflurane and halothane. Volatile liquids are administered as a vapour after vapourization in a device called vapourizer.

General anaesthesia consists of three phases: (a) Induction, (b) maintenance, and (c) recovery of anaesthesia.

Inhalational anaesthetic agents are mainly used for maintenance of anaesthesia. However, halothane and sevoflurane are also used for induction of anaesthesia, especially in the paediatric population.

Minimal Alveolar Concentration (MAC)

Minimum concentration of an anaesthetic agent at the alveolus, which produces a lack of reflex movement in 50% of non-paralysed subjects to skin incision.

For induction of anaesthesia, 2 to 3 MAC value of inhalation agent is required. MAC value 1 to 1.5 is adequate for the maintenance of anaesthesia.

AD_{95}: Median anaesthetic dose to obtund reflex movement in 95% of subjects. AD_{95} is about 1.5 times of MAC value (Table 35.1).

Table 35.1	Physical properties of inhalational anaesthetic agents			
Agent	**Molecular weight**	**Boiling point (°C)**	**MAC (%)**	**Meta-bolism (%)**
Nitrous oxide	44	-88.5	104	0.004
Desflurane	168	23.5	6.0	0.2
Halothane	197	50	0.75	20
Isoflurane	184.5	48.5	1.15	0.2
Sevoflurane	200	58.5	2.00	3

Mechanism of Action

- Inhalational agents act at multiple sites by more than one mechanism.
- Immobilization effect of the inhalational agent is determined at spinal cord level, whereas sedation, hypnosis and amnesia by inhalational agents involve supraspinal mechanisms.
- Inhalational anaesthetic agents enhance inhibitory synaptic transmission.

Systemic Effects of Inhalational Anaesthetic Agents

Central Nervous System

- **Cerebral metabolic oxygen requirement (CMRO$_2$):** There is a dose-dependent decrease in cerebral activity and reduction in oxygen demand by the brain.
- **Cerebral protection:** Isoflurane, sevoflurane and desflurane reduce CMRO$_2$ and thus protect the brain against ischaemic injury.
- **Intracranial pressure (ICP):** Inhalational anaesthetic agents cause cerebral vaso-dilatation and increase cerebral blood flow and may increase intracranial pressure.

Cardiovascular System

- **Cardiac output:** Isoflurane, desflurane and sevoflurane have minimum effect on cardiac output. Halothane depresses myocardium and thus reduces cardiac output.
- **Heart rate:** Isoflurane, desflurane and sevoflurane increase heart rate. Halothane causes depression of baroreceptor reflex and sinus node and may produce brady-cardia.
- **Mean arterial pressure:** All volatile anaesthetic agents produce a dose-dependent decrease in mean arterial pressure.
- **Systemic vascular resistance:** Isoflurane, desflurane and sevoflurane produce dose dependent reduction in systemic vascular resistance. Nitrous oxide and halothane have no effect.

Respiratory System

- **Breathing:** All inhalational anaesthetic agents produce rapid and shallow breathing during general anaesthesia. Ventilator response to hypoxia and hypercarbia is obtunded by these agents.
- **Airway reactivity:** All inhalational anaesthetic agents are bronchodilator. Isoflurane and desflurane cause irritation to the upper airway and may produce laryngospasm.

Liver

All inhalational anaesthetic agents cause some degree of hepatic dysfunction due to the reduction of hepatic blood flow and oxygen delivery. Repeated exposure of halothane in a genetically predisposed individual may produce halothane hepatitis.

Kidney

Inhalational anaesthetic agents cause a reduction in glomerular filtration rate and urine output due to a reduction in renal blood flow.

INTRAVENOUS ANAESTHETIC AGENTS

Intravenous anaesthetic agents are administered by intravenous route as an induction agent to induce general anaesthesia quickly and smoothly. Some of them may also be used for maintenance of anaesthesia either alone or in combination with other drugs. They are also used for sedation during regional anaesthesia, and at intensive care unit.

Properties of an Ideal Intravenous Anaesthetic Agent

- It should produce rapid induction and rapid recovery of anaesthesia.
- The subanaesthetic dose should produce sedation and analgesia.
- Minimal cardiovascular and respiratory depression.
- No toxic effect on other organs.
- No emetic effect, no pain at the site of injection and no histamine release.
- It should not cause a hypersensitivity reaction.

Commonly used Intravenous Anaesthetic Agents (Table 35.2)

Propofol: Propofol is an alkylphenol derivative. It produces rapid onset and recovery of anaesthesia. It acts on the β-subunit of the $GABA_A$ receptor and causes hyperpolarization by increasing chloride channel opening time.

Thiopentone sodium: It is ultrashort-acting barbiturate. It produces rapid onset and recovery of anaesthesia when used as a single dose, but repeated-dose prolongs the recovery from anaesthesia. It acts on $GABA_A$ and glycine receptors and increases channel opening time for chloride.

Midazolam: Midazolam belongs to the benzodiazepine group of the drug. Onset time of midazolam is slower than propofol and thiopentone. It acts on 'y' subunit of the $GABA_A$ receptor complex. It augments hyper-polarization by increasing the frequency of channel opening.

Ketamine: It is phencyclidine derivatives. It acts as an antagonist of the N-methyl D aspartate receptor. It produces dissociative anaesthesia. Muscle tone is maintained but there are profound analgesia and amnesia.

Etomidate: It is an imidazole derivative. It is preferred for induction of anaesthesia in patients with the compromised cardiovascular system. Although onset and recovery of anaesthesia are very fast following etomidate injection, adrenocortical suppression is the main limiting factor. It activates and modulates $β_2$ and $β_3$ subunits of $GABA_A$ receptors.

Dexmedetomidine: It is s-enantiomer of medetomidine, a selective $α_2$ adrenergic agonist. It produces sedation, sympatholysis, hypnosis and analgesia. It is used as premedicant and procedural sedation.

Table 35.2		Dosage and key points of commonly used intravenous anaesthetic agents		
S no.	IV anaesthetic agent	Commercially available preparation	Dose	Key points
1.	Propofol	1% propofol of 20, 50 and 100 ml ampoule/vial	Induction: 1–2.5 mg/kg Maintenance: 50–150 µg/kg/min Sedation: 25–75 µg/kg/min	Used for induction and maintenance of anaes-thesia (TIVA)
2.	Thiopentone sodium	The vial containing 500 mg powder, dissolve in water and prepare a 2.5% solution	Induction: 3–4 mg/kg Maintenance: 50–100 mg every 10–12 min (not preferred)	Used as an induction agent Not used for main-tenance of anaesthesia by continuous infusion
3.	Etomidate	Vial containing 20 mg/ 10 ml (0.2% solution)	Induction: 0.2–0.6 mg/kg	Maintain cardiovascular stability. Used as inducing agent in compromised cardiac patient
4.	Midazolam	1,3 and 5 ml ampoule of 1mg/ml and 5 mg/ml	Induction: 0.15–0.3 mg/kg Maintenance: 2 µg/kg/min Sedation: 2–5 µg/kg/min	Used as sedative. It pro-duces less cardiovascular and respiratory depression.
5.	Ketamine	Ampoule or vial containing 1%, 5% and 10% solution	Induction: 1–2 mg/kg Sedation and analgesia: 0.2–0.8 mg/kg Maintenance: 25–100 µg/kg/min	Produces amnesia and profound analgesia but no reflex suppression.

Pharmacological Effects

Table 35.3	Effects of intravenous anaesthetic agents on cardiovascular, respiratory and central nervous system							
S. no.	IV agents	Cardiovascular system		Respiratory system		Central nervous system		
		HR	MAP	Ventilation	Broncho-dilator	CBF	CMRO₂	ICP
1.	Thiopentone	↑↑	↓↓	↓↓↓	↓	↓↓↓	↓↓↓	↓↓↓
2.	Propofol	0	↓↓↓	↓↓↓	0	↓↓↓	↓↓↓	↓↓↓
3.	Etomidate	0	↓	↓	0	↓↓↓	↓↓↓	↓↓↓
4.	Ketamine	↑↑	↑↑	↓	↑↑↑	↑↑↑	↑	↑↑↑
	Benzodiazepine							
5.	Diazepam	0/↑	↓	↓↓	0	↓↓	↓↓	↓↓
6.	Lorazepam	0/↑	↓	↓↓	0	↓↓	↓↓	↓↓
7.	Midazolam	↑	↓↓	↓↓	0	↓↓	↓↓	↓↓
	Opioids							
8.	Pethidine	↑	0	↓↓↓	0/↓	↓	↓	↓
9.	Morphine	↓	0	↓↓↓	0/↓	↓	↓	↓
10.	Fentanyl	↓↓	↓/0	↓↓↓	0	↓	↓	↓
11.	Sufentanil	↓↓	↓/0	↓↓↓	0	↓	↓	↓
12.	Alfentanil	↓↓	↓	↓↓↓	0	↓	↓	↓
13.	Remifentanil	↓↓	↓	↓↓↓	0	↓	↓	↓

HR = heart rate, MAP= mean arterial pressure, CBF= cerebral blood flow, CMRO₂ = central oxygen consumption, ICP = intracranial pressure, 0 = no change, ↓, ↓↓, ↓↓↓ = mild, moderate and marked decrease, ↑,↑↑,↑↑↑ = mild, moderate, marked increase.

Adverse Effects

Table 35.4	Induction, recovery quality and adverse effects of intravenous anaesthetic agents		
S no.	Intravenous anaesthetic agents	Induction/recovery quality	Adverse effects/contraindications
1.	Thiopentone sodium	Fast onset but slow recovery especially after continuous infusion.	• Hypersensitivity • Extravasation cause tissue damage and ulcer **Contraindications** • Porphyria • Status asthmaticus
2.	Propofol	Fast onset and fast recovery	• Abnormal myoclonic movement • Pain on injection • Hypersensitivity
3.	Etomidate	Fast onset and fast recovery	• Adrenocortical suppression
4.	Ketamine	The slow onset and slow recovery, emergence common	**Contraindications** • Raised intracranial pressure • Penetrating eye injury
5.	Midazolam	The slow onset and slow recovery	• Nausea-vomiting· • Respiratory depression

ANALGESICS

All patients need analgesics during surgery and postoperative period for relief from the surgical pain. Opioids and nonsteroidal anti-inflammatory drugs are used to provide pain relief during the perioperative period.

Opioids are narcotic analgesics acting on opioid receptors; Mu, Kappa and Delta. They are present at presynaptic and postsynaptic sites in the brain, spinal cord and peripheral tissue. They produce analgesia, sedation and euphoria. Opioid overdose may cause respiratory depression which can be treated by an opioid antagonist such as naloxone.

NSAIDs act by inhibition of COX enzyme and produce analgesia, anti-inflammation and antipyretic effects. It may be nonspecific COX inhibitors such as aspirin, paracetamol, ibuprofen or COX-2 inhibitors. Potential side effects are gastric ulceration, renal dysfunction and inhibition of platelet aggregation.

NEUROMUSCULAR BLOCKING AGENTS

Neuromuscular blocking agents are commonly known as muscle relaxants, used to achieve muscular relaxation for tracheal intubation, control ventilation and optimize surgical operating conditions (Tables 35.5 and 35.6).

Mechanism of Action

- Neuromuscular blocking agents interrupt the transmission of nerve impulses at the neuromuscular junction. They are positively charged quaternary ammonium compound and combine with α subunit of nicotinic receptors.
- Depolarization muscle relaxant suxamethonium acts on the receptor and produces depolarization for a longer period and makes receptors unresponsive to subsequent stimulation.
- Non-depolarization muscle relaxants compete with acetylcholine, occupy receptor binding site, interrupt the transmission of nerve impulse and thus prevent contraction of muscles.

Classification of Neuromuscular Blocking Agents

- Depolarizing muscle relaxants
  - Suxamethonium
- Nondepolarizing muscle relaxants
  - Atracurium
  - Cis-atracurium
  - Doxacurium
  - Pancuronium

Table 35.5	Pharmacodynamics of muscle relaxants			
Muscle relaxants	ED_{95} (mg/kg)	Intubating dose (mg/kg)	Onset time (sec)	Duration of action (min)
Suxamethonium	0.3	1.0	60	10
Atracurium	0.23	0.5	110	40
Cis-atracurium	0.05	0.15	150	45
Doxacurium	0.025	0.05	250	80
Pancuronium	0.07	0.1	220	75
Pipecuronium	0.045	0.08	300	95
Rocuronium	0.3	0.6	75	30
Vecuronium	0.05	0.1	180	30

ED_{95} mean dose of muscle relaxant that depresses twitch height by 95%. Intubation dose is usually $2 \times ED_{95}$ or $3 \times ED_{95}$.

Table 35.6	Excretion of muscle relaxants	
Muscle relaxants	Urinary excretion (%)	Biliary excretion (%)
Atracurium	10	–
Cis-atracurium	15	–
Doxacurium	30	–
Pancuronium	40	10
Pipecuronium	38	2
Rocuronium	10	55
Vecuronium	15	40

- Pipecuronium
- Rocuronium
- Vecuronium
- D-Tubocurarine

Side Effects of Muscle Relaxants

Common side effects of suxamethonium include sinus bradycardia, ventricular arrhythmias, hyperkalaemia, and increased intragastric pressure, intracranial, intraocular pressure. Myalgia is common following suxamethonium injection.

The hypersensitive reaction may occur following non-depolarizing muscle relaxants. Cardiovascular side effects are due to histamine release, ganglionic effects, vagolytic action or sympathetic stimulation (Table 35.7).

Antagonism of Neuromuscular Block

At the end of the surgical procedure, residual neuromuscular blockade is reversed by anticholinesterase, neostigmine. It inhibits acetylcholinesterase, which is responsible for rapid hydrolysis of acetylcholine at the neuromuscular junction. As a result, the concentration of acetylcholine increases at the neuromuscular junction and overcome the effects of neuromuscular blockers. The dose of neostigmine is 2.5 mg with 1 mg atropine or 0.5 mg glycopyrrolate. Maximum dose of neostigmine is 5 mg.

LOCAL ANAESTHETIC AGENTS

Local anaesthetic agents cause reversible inhibition of nerve conduction. They interrupt neuronal transmission by preventing the passage of sodium ions through selective sodium channels of nerve membrane. In this way, they prevent depolarization, generation of action potential and nerve conduction. Transmission of autonomic, sensory and motor impulses is prevented on the dose-dependent manner and there is a complete recovery of nerve transmission without any residual effect.

Classification of Local Anaesthetics

- Ester-linked local anaesthetics
  - Procaine
  - Chloroprocaine

Table 35.7	Cardiovascular side effects			
Muscle relaxants	Histamine release	Ganglionic effects	Vagolytic activity	Sympathetic stimulation
Suxamethonium	+	Stimulation	0	0
Atracurium	+	0	0	0
Cis-atracurium	0	0	0	0
Pancuronium	0	0	+	+
Pipecuronium	0	0	0	0
Rocuronium	0	0	±	0
Vecuronium	0	0	0	0

Table 35.8	Local anaesthetics with different concentrations, dosage and use in clinical practice			
Agents	**Concentrations**	**Maximum safe dose (mg/kg)**	**Duration of action**	**Uses in a different technique of neuronal blocks**
Lignocaine	0.5%, 1%, 1.5%, 2%, 4%, 5% and 10%	4.5 (without adrenaline) 7 (with adrenaline)	Medium	Spinal, epidural, peripheral nerve blocks, topical including spray, infiltration and intravenous regional anaesthesia
Prilocaine	0.5%, 2%	8	Medium	EMLA cream as topical anaesthesia
Bupivacaine	0.25%, 0.5%	3	Long	Spinal, epidural, infiltration and peripheral nerve blocks
Levobupivacaine	0.15%, 0.5% and 0.75%	3	Long	Epidural, peripheral nerve blocks
Ropivacaine	0.2%, 0.5% and 0.75%	3	Long	Spinal, epidural, infiltration and peripheral nerve blocks

- Tetracaine
- Amide linked local anaesthetics
  - Lignocaine
  - Prilocaine
  - Bupivacaine
  - Levobupivacaine
  - Ropivacaine
  - Mepivacaine

Local anaesthetic agents commonly used for blocking the nerve conduction are lignocaine, bupivacaine, levobupivacaine and ropivacaine (Table 35.8).

Toxicity of Local Anaesthetics

Central nervous system: Toxicity is manifested as circumoral numbness, metallic taste, tinnitus, dizziness, confusion and convulsion.

Cardiovascular system: Toxicity is initially manifested as tachycardia and high blood pressure followed by hypotension, brady-cardia, myocardial depression, conduction abnormalities, ventricular arrhythmias and finally cardiac arrest.

Newer local anaesthetic agents, levobupivacaine and ropivacaine, are safer than bupivacaine but not free from cardiac and CNS toxicity with a higher dosage.

Treatment

- Maintain airway and oxygen therapy.
- Control convulsion with benzodiazepine, thiopentone or propofol.
- CPR, if cardiac arrest.
- Intralipid 20%, 1.5 ml/kg bolus, followed by 15 ml/kg/hour

Allergic Reaction

Allergy to local anaesthetics is rare, but it may manifest as bronchospasm, urticaria or angioneurotic oedema.

CHAPTER 36

Common Perioperative Complications

Over recent years, perioperative and anaesthetic complications have been decreased. It is 1 in 5 for minor complications, 1 in 100 for major complications and 1 in 1,00,000 for deaths.

COMMON RESPIRATORY COMPLICATIONS

Airway Obstruction

Airway obstruction is a medical emergency that may occur before, during and after anaesthesia. Diagnosis and management are often done simultaneously in patients with airway obstruction. Signs and symptoms of airway obstruction are as follows.

- **Patient with spontaneous ventilation:**
  - Retraction of intercostals, supraclavicular and abdominal muscles
  - Use of accessory muscles of respiration and movements of ala nasi
  - Diminished or absent breath sound
  - Noisy breathing, if the obstruction is partial
  - Cyanosis, restlessness, sweating, tachycardia and other features of hypoxia and hypercarbia.
- **Patient on artificial ventilation:**
  - Little or no movement of the thorax or abdominal wall
  - Diminished or absent breath sound

  - High lung inflation pressure
  - Features of hypoxia and hypercarbia

Causes of Airway Obstruction in the Perioperative Period

- Most commonly due to the tongue falling back against the posterior pharyngeal wall.
- Other causes include:
  - Secretion, blood or vomits in airway
  - Retained throat pack
  - Laryngospasm, glottis oedema

Treatment

- Oxygen supplementation.
- Corrective measures to remove the cause of obstruction:
  - Posterior displacement of the tongue can be prevented by jaw thrust (anterior displacement) and head tilt manoeuvre.
  - Oropharyngeal and nasopharyngeal airways are equally effective in maintaining clear upper airway.
  - Vomitus, blood or secretions may be removed from upper airway by using a suction machine.
  - Laryngospasm usually occurs due to surgical manipulation at the lighter plane of anaesthesia. Therefore, treatment consists of:

- Cessation of surgical stimulation,
- Increasing depth of anaesthesia, and
- Gentle positive airway pressure with a higher percentage of oxygen at inspired gases.
  - Sometime anaesthesiologists use a small dosage of short-acting muscle relaxant in refractory cases of laryngospasm.

Hypoventilation

- Hypoventilation or inadequate ventilation is very common following general anaesthesia. It causes accumulation of carbon dioxide and raised $PaCO_2$ level.
- Signs and symptoms of hypoventilation include slow respiratory rate or tachypnoea with shallow respiration or laboured breathing.
- Features of hypercapnia such as tachycardia, hypertension, arrhythmia, sweating and generalized oozing from the wound may be present.
- Hypoventilation in the postoperative period is very common due to residual effects of anaesthetic agents. Anaesthesiologist should identify the causative agent and use appropriate antidotes to reverse the effect and treat hypoventilation.
- Support or control ventilation as a supportive measure to treat hypercapnia.

Hypoxaemia

- Hypoxaemia means an abnormally low level of oxygen in the blood. It may cause tissue hypoxia as the blood is unable to supply enough oxygen to the body.
- Mild to moderate hypoxaemia is very common in patients recovering from general anaesthesia. Persistent hypoxaemia causes sympathetic stimulation and characterized by tachycardia, restlessness, agitation, irregular pulse rate/heart rate and, cyanosis (bluish discolouration of the mucous membrane).

- Postoperative hypoxaemia is usually caused by hypoventilation with or without obstruction. Therefore, the patient should be assessed for upper airway obstruction and/or hypoventilation.
- Treatment of hypoxaemia includes oxygen therapy with or without positive airway pressure (CPAP) and relief of any existing airway obstruction.

CIRCULATORY COMPLICATIONS

The common circulatory complications in the perioperative period are hypotension, hypertension and dysrhythmias.

Hypotension

Hypotension or fall in systemic blood pressure leads to inadequate delivery of oxygen and nutrients at the cellular level. It may be due to hypovolaemia, left ventricular dysfunction or excessive arterial vasodilatation.

Causes of Hypotension

- Hypovolaemia or intravascular volume depletion
  - Surgical bleeding
  - Gastrointestinal losses
  - Ongoing third space loss
  - Loss due to increased capillary permeability
    - Burn
    - Sepsis
- Decreased cardiac output due to left ventricular dysfunction
  - Perioperative myocardial ischaemia or infarction
  - Cardiac dysrhythmias
  - Pre-existing cardiac conditions cause to fall in cardiac output
- Excessive arterial vasodilatation
  - Sepsis
  - After central neuraxial block (spinal and epidural anaesthesia)
  - Allergic or anaphylactic reactions

Treatment

- Mild hypotension is common and does not require intensive treatment.
- If fall in blood pressure is more than 20–30% from baseline, the anaesthesiologist must be informed.
- Hypovolaemia is the commonest cause and hence bolus of intravenous fluid (250–500 ml crystalloid or 100–250 ml colloid) is administered. Positive response in terms of rise in blood pressure confirms hypovolemia and further volume replacement is indicated.
- Anaesthesiologist may use vasopressor or inotrope in case of severe hypotension especially when sepsis is suspected.
- Anaesthesiologist also assesses for any signs of cardiac dysfunction and takes appropriate measures.

Hypertension

- Patients with a history of essential hypertension are at increased risk for hypertension in the perioperative period. Other factors which may cause hypertension especially in the postoperative period are a pain, emergence excitement, urinary retention and nausea-vomiting.
- The rise in blood pressure more than 20–30% of the baseline are associated with adverse effects such as myocardial ischaemia, excessive bleeding, etc.
- On duty doctor must be informed for further evaluation of cause and management.

Cardiac Dysrhythmias

- The hypoventilation associated with hypoxaemia and/or hypercarbia is the commonest cause of cardiac dysrhythmias during the perioperative period. It may be due to metabolic abnormalities, preoperative cardiac or pulmonary disease.
- Any type of dysrhythmias noticed in ECG or heartbeat must be recorded and reported to anaesthesiologist for prompt intervention.

NEUROLOGICAL COMPLICATIONS

Postoperative Emergence Excitement/Agitation

- It is a transitional confusion state of the patient during emergence from general anaesthesia. It is more common in children than in adult.
- It usually occurs within 10 minutes after recovery from anaesthesia and associated with severe restlessness, agitation and excitement.
- It commonly occurs in patients who rapidly recover from anaesthesia. Other causative factors are postoperative pain, preoperative anxiety, type of surgery and type of anaesthetic drugs used.
- Preventive measures include:
  - Reduction of preoperative anxiety
  - Reduction of postoperative pain
  - Provision of the stress-free environment during recovery

Treatment

- Identification and management of causative factors.
- Inform anaesthesiologist for further management by using drugs such as midazolam, clonidine or dexmedetomidine.

Seizures

- Seizures are caused due to paroxysmal discharges from abnormally excitable neuronal foci. They can be tonic-clonic, generalized seizures or partial focal motor seizures.
- It may be due to underlying neurological disorders (head injury, brain tumour, etc.) or associated with toxicity of certain anaesthetic agents.
- Sometimes, unintentional withdrawal of anticonvulsant agent in the perioperative

period may precipitate seizures in patients on the anticonvulsant agent.

- Preventive measures include:
  - Identification of patients with pre-existing seizure disorders.
  - Continue anticonvulsant agent in the perioperative period.

Treatment

- Prevention of traumatic injury during seizures
- Secure airway
- Oxygen supplementation
- Report on-duty doctor for control of seizures.

CHAPTER 37

Cardiopulmonary Resuscitation

Cardiopulmonary resuscitation (CPR) or emergency cardiac care should be initiated immediately following a cardiac and respiratory arrest. CPR should also be considered, if any individual is unable to oxygenate or perfuse vital organs.

Cardiac arrest is diagnosed, if there are no signs of life and the individual is not breathing normally. Gasping type of respiration may be seen transiently in 40% of individuals following cardiac arrest.

The success of resuscitation depends upon the chain of survival that consists of: Call for help → initiation of basic life support (BLS) and early defibrillation → optimum post-resuscitation care (Fig. 37.1).

BASIC LIFE SUPPORT

Basic life support must be initiated to all patients who are unresponsive and not breathing normally. Basic life support consists of circulation, airway, breathing and as early as possible defibrillation (CABDs). The main steps of basic life support are given in Fig. 37.2.

During CPR

- Attempt to place, confirm and secure airway
- Attempt to establish IV access
- Patients with VT/VF refractory to initial shocks

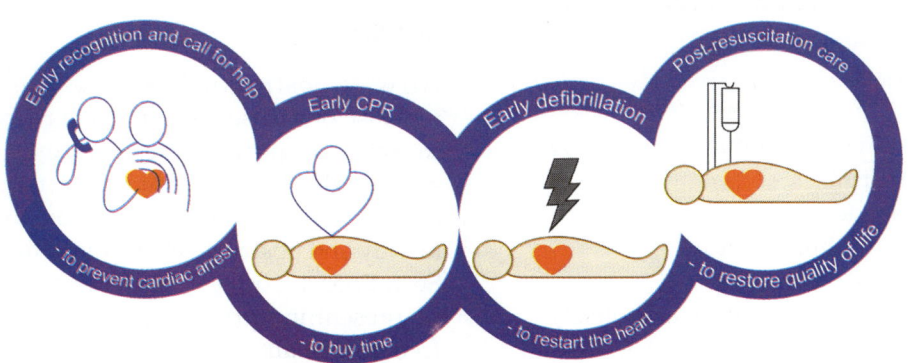

Fig. 37.1: Chain of survival

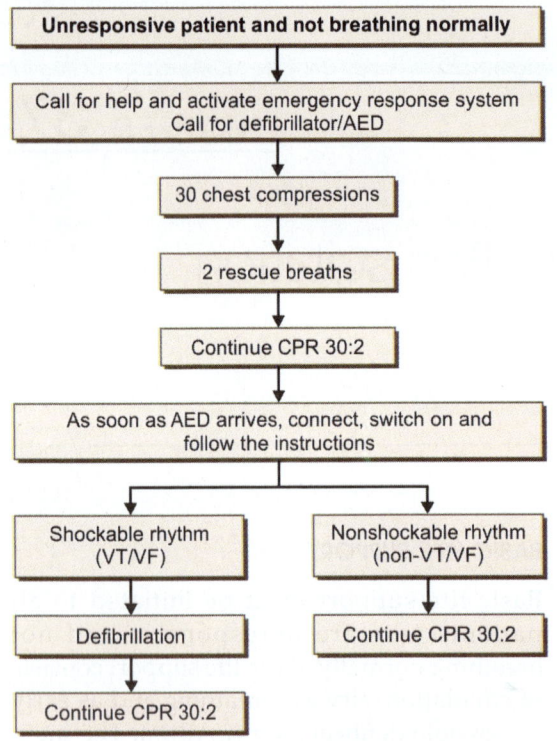

Fig. 37.2: Adult basic life support algorithm

- Epinephrine 1 mg IV every 3–5 minutes
  or
- Vasopressin 40 U IV single dose
- Patients with non-shockable (non-VT/VF) rhythms
  - Epinephrine 1 mg IV every 3–5 minutes
- Search and correct reversible causes.

Reversible Causes of Cardiac Arrest

- Hypovolaemia
- Hypoxia
- Hydrogen ion acidosis
- Hypo-/hyperkalaemia
- Hypothermia
- Tamponade (cardiac)
- Tension (pneumothorax)
- Thrombosis, coronary
- Thrombosis (pulmonary embolism)
- Tablets, drugs, poisons

CHEST COMPRESSION

- Chest compressions should be immediately initiated on the discovery of a suspected cardiac arrest.
- Chest compressions force the blood to flow and supply oxygen and nutrients to vital organs especially the brain by increasing intrathoracic pressure or by directly compressing the heart.

Steps of Chest Compression

- The victim of cardiac arrest should be on a firm surface.
- Compress the lower half of sternum by placing the heel of one hand on the sternum, at the levels of nipples. The heel of the other hand should be placed over first hand and interlock the fingers (Fig: 37.3).
- Shoulder of the rescuer should be positioned directly over the victim, with elbow locked.
- Sternal depression during chest compression should be 5–6 cm or more.
- Press hard and fast.
- Allow for full chest recoil after each compression.
- Compression should be given at a rate of 100 to 120 per minute without pause for ventilation.
- Allow for only minimal interruptions to chest compressions (Fig. 37.3).

AIRWAY

Airway obstruction is very common in unconscious patients, due to the relaxation of muscles supporting the mandible, tongue, and epiglottis. The base of the tongue and epiglottis fall back posterior on the upper airway and obstruct gas flow into the trachea. Secretions, blood or other foreign bodies may be present in upper airway and obstruct the free flow of air.

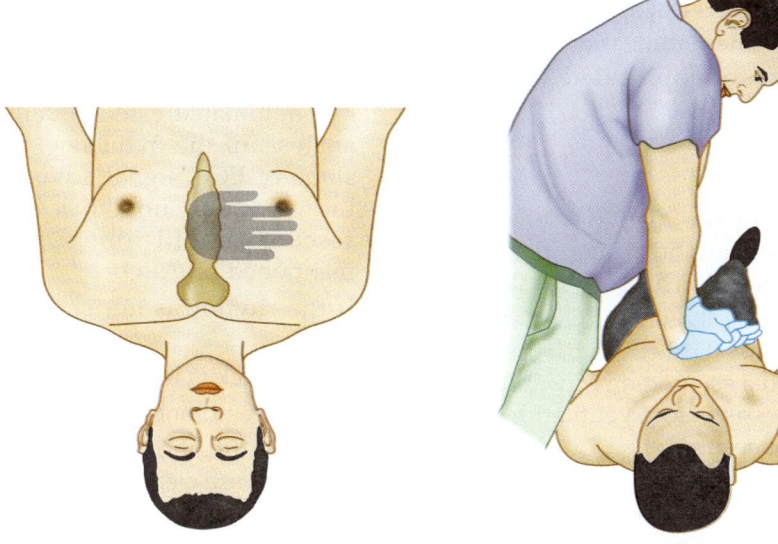

Fig. 37.3: Chest compression

Establishment of the Clear Upper Airway

- **Triple manoeuvre:** Head tilt, chin lift, and jaw thrust manoeuvre to reposition tongue and epiglottis to its normal position and clear upper airway.
  - Head tilt-chin lift manoeuvre (when cervical spine injury has been excluded:
    - Place the palm on the forehead of the patient and apply pressure to tilt the head backward.
    - Place the fingers of another hand under the mental protuberance of the chin and pull the chin forward and cephalic (Fig: 37.4).

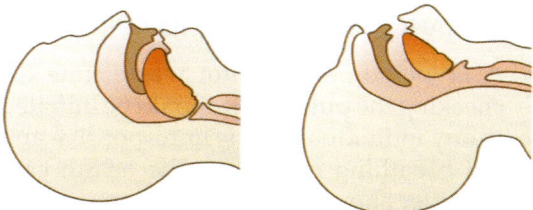

Fig. 37.4: Clear upper airway

  - Jaw thrust manoeuvre (when cervical spine injury has not been ruled out):
    - Place fingers of both hands on the lower rami of the jaw.
    - Apply anterior pressure to advance jaw forward.
- Removal of a foreign body by suction machine, finger sweep or Magill forceps under direct vision.
- Clear airway by placing oropharyngeal or nasopharyngeal airway into the upper airway.
- Combitube or LMA can be used by experts for securing the airway.

Signs of Cervical Spine Injury

- Significant distracting injury in and around the neck'.
- Spinal pain with or without neurological signs or symptoms.
- Patient with a reduced level of consciousness

- **Management:** Prevention of movement at the level of the cervical spine by:
  - Manual in-line stabilization (MILS)
  - Application of appropriate size of the semi-rigid collar.

BREATHING

If, after opening the airway, there is no evidence of adequate breathing, the rescuer should assist ventilation by a bag-mask device.

- Rescue breathing should deliver 400–700 ml of tidal volume, 8–10 times per minute in an adult with a secured airway and a ratio of 30 compressions to 2 ventilations, if the airway is not secured.
- The breath should be delivered slowly over a period of 2 seconds with a smaller tidal volume to minimize adverse effects on cardiac preload.
- Adequacy of ventilation is assessed by observation of chest wall movement and auscultation of breath sound.
- Compression should not be suspended to permit ventilation unless it is not possible to ventilation during compressions.
- Supplemental oxygen preferably 100% should be used, if available.

DEFIBRILLATION

Aim of defibrillation is to deliver sufficient transmyocardial current to depolarize a critical mass of myocardium allowing restoration of synchronized electrical activity.

Defibrillation within three minutes after cardiac arrest is the major determinant of successful resuscitation. Therefore, early defibrillation is the priority.

- Defibrillation is done by an automated external defibrillator. Attach and use AED as soon as available.
- Apply the pads to the chest wall of the victim according to the pictures on the back of the pads. One pad is placed on the right side of the chest, just below the clavicle.

Another pad is placed on the lower left side of the chest.

- Connect the pads to the AED and turn on the AED.
- The automated external defibrillator, after analysis of the frequency, amplitude and slope of ECG signal advise either 'shock indicated' or 'no shock indicated'. The rescuer should follow the instruction mentioned by AED.
- If the rhythm is not shockable, continue CPR.
- If the shock is indicated:
  - Assure no one is touching the patient.
  - Press the shock button when the providers are clear of the victim.
  - Resume CPR beginning with compressions immediately after each shock.
  - Minimize interruptions in chest compressions before and aftershock.

POST-CARDIAC ARREST MANAGEMENT

Following the return of spontaneous circulation (ROSC):

- Shift the victim to an intensive care unit as early as possible for further management.
- Optimize ventilation and oxygenation with a goal to maintain oxygen saturation ≥94%.
- Treat hypotension with intravenous fluid and vasopressors.
- Consider targeted temperature management between 32 and 36°C.
- Find out the cause of cardiac arrest and consider treating causative factors such as urgent coronary artery catheterization.

IMPORTANT POINTS RELATED TO CPR

- A layperson should not waste time for checking the pulse. CPR should be initiated in any individual who is unresponsive and not breathing normally. The health care provider should assess for the presence or absence of a carotid pulse.

- Chest compression without ventilation may be as effective as compression with ventilation for the first several minutes.
- However, survival is greater in hypoxic related arrest when rescue breaths are also given.
- Uninterrupted high-quality chest compressions, minimizing interruption time of compression and pre-shock pause are important determining factors for the outcome of CPR.
- A single resuscitative shock should be delivered at the earlier possible opportunity after recognition of cardiac arrest and immediately followed by the resumption of chest compression.
- The rules of tens and multiples:
  - Less than 10 seconds to check for pulse.
  - Less than 10 seconds to place and secure the airway.
  - Target chest compression adequacy.
    - To maintain end-tidal carbon dioxide greater than 10 mm Hg.
    - To maintain arterial diastolic blood pressure greater than 20 mm Hg.
    - To maintain central venous oxygen saturation greater than 30 mm Hg.

CHAPTER 38

Mass Casualty and Triage

Emergency: Incidence where the health status of an individual demands for urgent action is called an emergency. Example: Patient with motorbike accident, stroke, angina, etc.

Mass casualty: Large number of casualties in a short period that initially exceeds the local logistic support capabilities. Example: Train collision, airplane crash, mass poisoning, etc.

Disaster: Large number of casualties and destroyed infrastructure that exceeds local/regional response capabilities. National forces are needed to solve the problem. Example: Earthquake, cyclone, chemical or nuclear disaster, etc.

Duty of the first team at the scene: First team reaches the scene must conduct:

- A quick assessment of the scene including hazards, if any.
- Assessment of the possible number of victims.
- Communicate to the control room for activation and early dispatch of emergency medical service. EMS system deploys logistics, coordinates and communicates with the team working at the site of the mass casualty incident.

TRIAGE SYSTEM

Triage is the process of determining the priority of the patient's treatment based on the severity of their condition. This offers patient treatment more rational when resources are insufficient for all to be treated immediately.

Principles of Triage

- Do the greatest good to the greatest number of people.
- Deploy the most efficient use of available resources.
- Treat as many as possible who have a chance of survival by shifting the patients away from the incident toward resources that offer more comprehensive care.
- Treatment during triage is minimal.
- Triage is a dynamic process because patients' clinical status may change and may switch over from one category to another.

START Triage

Simple triage and rapid treatment (START) is the most widely used triage system. First responders divide all the injured victims into four categories based on the severity of the injury and shift them to a designated collection point (Fig. 38.1).

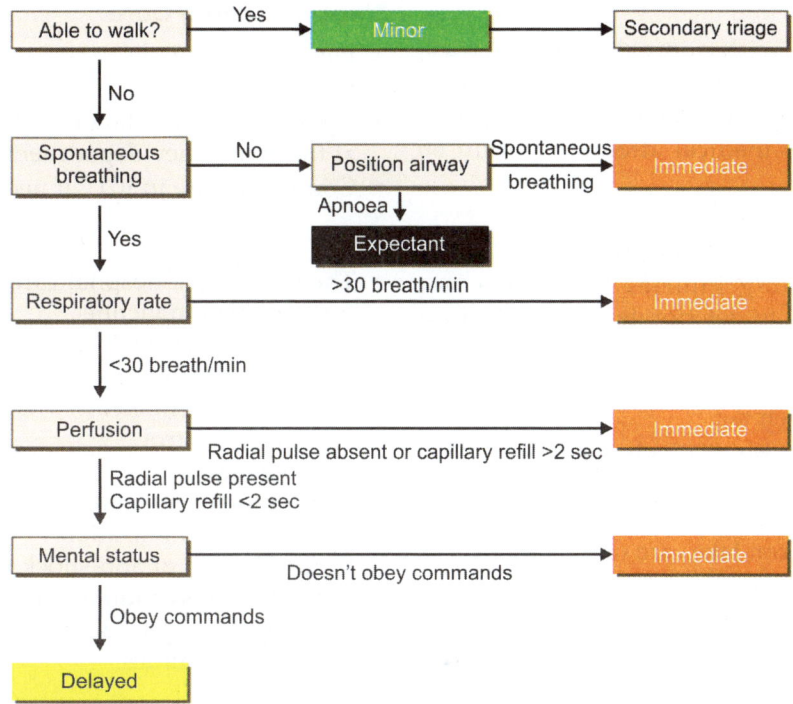

Fig. 38.1: START triage

- **Black** (deceased/expectant): Injuries incompatible with life or without spontaneous respiration should not be moved forward to the collection point.
- **Red** (immediate): Severe injuries but high potential for survival with treatment are shifted to collection point first.
- **Yellow** (delayed): Serious injuries but not immediately life-threatening.
- **Green** (walking wounded): Minor injuries.

Implementation of Triage

- Triage may be done by giving triage tags (black, red, yellow or green) to all patients or by physically sorting patients into different designated areas for different categories of patients.
- Ask the patients to move to a designated area, who can walk and level them green.
- Assess all non-ambulatory victims.

- Victims who are not breathing even after maintaining the clear upper airway are assigned a black tag.
- A red tag is assigned to the following patients:
  - Respiratory rate of more than 30.
  - Absent radial pulse or capillary refill more than 2 seconds.
  - Unable to follow simple commands.
- The yellow tag is assigned to the rest of the patients.

Triage Categories

- **Expectant:** Black tag
  - Victims unlike to survive due to the severity of injuries and level of available care.
  - Palliative care and pain relief should be provided.

- **Immediate:** Red tag
  - Victims with compromised airway, breathing, and circulation
  - Immediate intervention and transport
  - Requires medical attention within 60 minutes
- **Delayed:** Yellow tag
  - Victims with serious and potentially life-threatening injuries but status not expected to deteriorate during the next few hours.
  - Transport of patients can be delayed
- **Minor:** Green tag
  - Victims with relatively minor injuries
  - Status is unlikely to deteriorate over the next few days
  - Patients can take care of him/her.

Jump START

Jump START is a modification of the START system. It is used in children up to 8 years of age. If age is not known, then the presence of underarm hair in males and breast development in females is considered as adult.

Modifications are as follows:

- All apnoeic children with a pulse are given 5 rescue breaths; if no response, assigned a black tag.
- Abnormal respiratory rate is either less than 15 or more than 45.
- Neurological assessment is done by AVPU (alert, respond to verbal stimuli, respond to painful stimuli and unresponsive). Unresponsive patients and patients responding to painful stimuli are assigned a red tag.

Primary Care of Trauma Victims

Early intervention improves the prognosis of trauma victims. The first sixty minutes after the accident is called 'Golden Hour'. Therefore, optimum pre-hospital care of trauma victims by health care provider plays a crucial role in determining the outcome of the patient.

Steps of Trauma Care

- Early pre-hospital care
- Early transport
- Aggressive resuscitation and interventions at the emergency department
- Continued care in ICU, if needed.

Pre-Hospital Care

- The goal of pre-hospital care is to prevent further harm to victims.
- Pre-hospital care includes a primary survey for the detection of obvious injuries and limited interventions.
  - Airway control
  - Oxygenation and ventilation support
  - Haemorrhage control
  - Spinal immobilization
  - Application of anti-shock trousers
  - Intravenous cannulations, if time allows.
  - Rapid transport to centres with appropriate facilities.

A. Airway Management

- Look for unobstructed normal respiration.
- Signs of airway obstruction are indrawing of the chest wall, use of accessory muscles, noisy breathing and presence of secretions or foreign materials in the upper airway.
- The clear airway can be achieved by:
  - The triple manoeuvre consists of head tilt, chin lift, and jaw thrust. Neck movement should be avoided in all suspected cases of cervical injury.
  - Remove foreign body and secretions from upper airway by suctions.
  - Insert oropharyngeal, nasopharyngeal airway or LMA.

Cervical spine protection

- Suspect cervical spine injury in patients with:
  - Multiple trauma
  - Blunt injury above the clavicle
  - Neck pain with or without neurological deficit
  - Unconscious patients

- Immobilize cervical spine by:
  - Manual in-line stabilization by holding the angles of the jaw from both hands and maintain constant traction from the head end side.
  - Placement of cervical collar

B. Breathing

- **Assessment:** Look for;
  - Increased respiratory rate
  - Cyanosis
  - Use of accessory muscles
  - Presence of any penetrating injury
  - Frail chest
- **Management:**
  - Oxygen therapy
  - Support ventilation

C. Circulation

- Assess for features of hypovolaemia:
  - Pulse rate more than 120/minute
  - Systolic blood pressure less than 80 mm Hg
  - Poor capillary refill
  - Cold clammy extremities
  - Altered consciousness

- **Management:**
  - Intravenous warm fluids (crystalloids) infusion up to 2 litres or 20 ml kg^{-1}.
  - Arrest bleeding by direct local pressure especially at extremities.
  - Warm blood and blood products transfusion
  - Damage control surgery

D. Disability

- Rapid neurological assessment by AVPU
  - A—Alert: CGS—14–15
  - V—Verbal stimulation respond: GCS—9–13
  - P—Respond to pain only: GCS—4–8
  - U—Unresponsive: GCS—3

E. Exposure and Assess for Injury All Over the Body

Environment: warm to prevent hypothermia

Endpoint of Resuscitation

- Stable haemodynamic status without any inotropic support.
- Maintaining oxygen saturation within an acceptable level.
- Normal body temperature
- Urine output >1 ml/kg/hour
- No coagulopathy

CHAPTER **39**

Operation Theatre Equipment

OPERATION THEATRE TABLE

It is a specialized table on which a patient is placed for a surgical procedure in operation theatre.

Parts of OT Table

* Base
* Column
* Top
* Attachments

Base

It is manually or electrically operated unit which can increase or decrease the height of the table.

Column

It is the middle portion of the table connecting the top and the base. The design of the column allows the tabletop to move in different directions.

Top

* It is the upper part of the table and made of a radiolucent material.
* It has different segments for resting leg, trunk and head and can bend according to the position of the body required for operation.

* The top is covered with a soft radiolucent pad to avoid pressure sore.
* In the modern OT table, the tabletop can be detached from the main unit and can be used for transport of the patient from one place to another (Fig. 39.1).

Attachments

* **Hand support:** Here both upper extremities are supported in a platform useful for intravenous fluid therapy, monitoring of vitals and operation in upper limbs.

* **Foot and leg support:** Two vertical metal bars are attached for leg support in the lithotomy position of the patient.

* **Fracture table:** This is an operation theatre table with a special attachment used for orthopaedic operations in hips and lower limbs. In this fracture table, the lower extremities are supported on foot piece and horizontal telescopic bars. One small vertical well-padded radiolucent pillar is attached in the caudal end of the table pressing perineum to allow longitudinal traction to the lower limbs.

* **Other attachments:** Apart from the above attachments, fluid stand, pelvic support guard in the lateral position of patient, screen stand to isolate head-end of table are

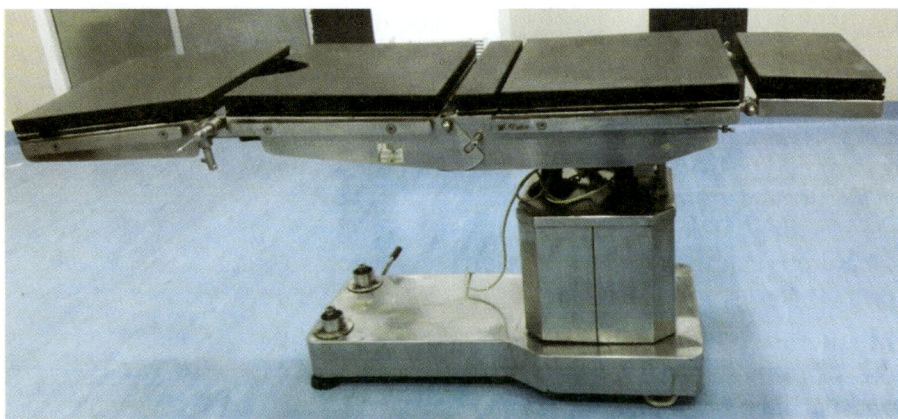

Fig. 39.1: Operation theatre table

also attached to main OT table as per the necessity of operation.

Uses

Patients are placed on the operation theatre table:

- For any surgical procedure
- For examination of the patient under anaesthesia
- For the application of plaster in a patient.

OT CEILING LIGHT

Ceiling light or surgical light is an illumination system which helps to visualize the objects in the operative field during the operation of a patient. It is designed in a way that does not radiate excessive heat on the operative field including patient. The colour of the light is very soothing and has daylight character for better visualization of different tissues in the operative field. Source of surgical lights may be Halogen lamps or LEDs.

Features

- Multiple lamps are mounted in the single or double dome which is suspended from the ceiling with the help of an arm. The modern surgical light system has a lightweight and can move in various directions.
- There is an autoclavable and detachable handle in the centre of the dome and the surgeon can adjust the focus of the light as required during operation (Fig. 39.2).

Uses

- To see the operative field properly during any surgical procedure in the operation room.
- To see the parts of the body or its cavity properly for diagnostic purposes (rectal or vaginal examination).

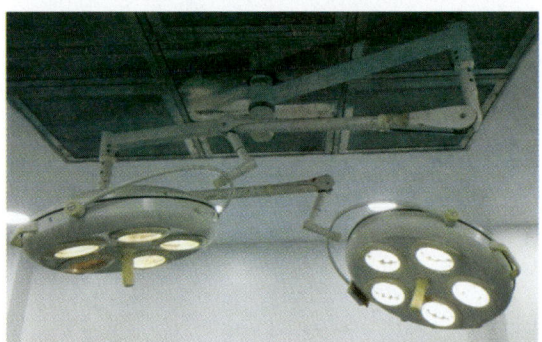

Fig. 39.2: OT light

ELECTROCAUTERY MACHINE

It is an electrosurgical machine used to arrest bleeding and to cut tissues in a surgical procedure. From this machine, high-frequency alternating current (HFAC) passes to the body tissue via a sterilized cord and produces heat to coagulate bleeding vessels and cut tissues without bleeding. There are two types of diathermy—unipolar and bipolar.

Unipolar diathermy: Current (HFAC) from machine passes to the body via a cord and returns to the machine via a patient return pad (touching the body of the patient). One pad with a cord is required which will connect body of the patient and machine.

Bipolar diathermy: Here both active and return electrodes are tips of the forceps. The current HFAC from machine passes through the bipolar forceps tip and the grasped tissue of the patient and then to the machine. There is no need to use a patient return pad to complete the circuit (Fig. 39.3).

Uses

- To stop bleeding from blood vessels during operation.
- To dissect soft tissue where too much bleeding is expected.

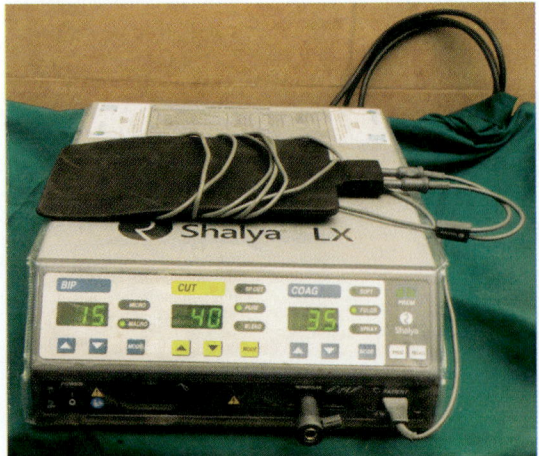

Fig. 39.3: Diathermy

SUCTION MACHINE

It is a motorized device where negative pressure is created and through a tube, the liquid materials of the body are sucked into the bottle attached to the machine (Fig. 39.4).

Features

- Suction machine
- Suction bottle
- Suction pipe

Uses

- To suck blood or blood mixed fluid in the operative field.
- To suck any secretion from the body especially from the mouth in an unconscious or anesthetized patient.

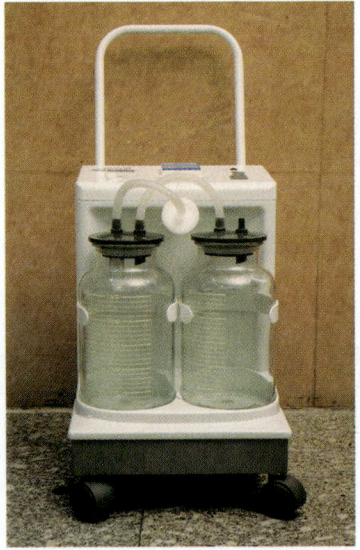

Fig. 39.4: Suction machine

TOURNIQUET

Surgical tourniquet system is a compressive device to prevent blood flow to the limbs and to create a bloodless field. The bloodless field helps to reduce blood loss and produces better visualization of tissues during surgery. It is important particularly in orthopaedic and plastic surgery of the limbs (Fig. 39.5).

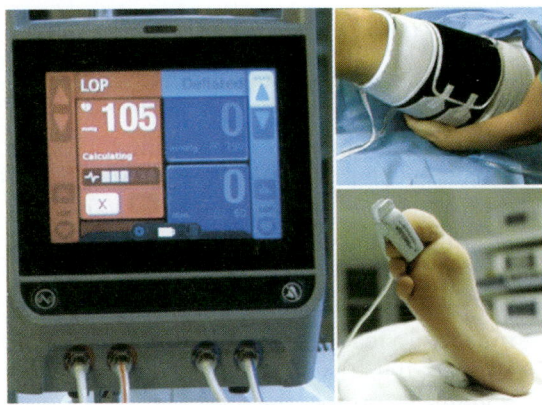

Fig. 39.5: Tourniquet

Types

- Esmarch rubber bandage
- Pneumatic tourniquet (electronic tourniquet)

Esmarch Rubber Bandage

It is a piece of rubber bandage measuring about 4 feet in length and 3 to 6 inches in breadth. It is applied over different parts of the limbs with pressure to occlude blood vessels. Before application, the limb is elevated and exsanguination of blood from the limb is done with one piece of Esmarch's bandage. Then the desired site is wrapped with a layer of cotton and the other piece of bandage is applied over the cotton wrapped area with pressure manually just to occlude the blood vessels of the limb.

Pneumatic Tourniquet

In the pneumatic tourniquet system, the blood vessels are occluded by external air pressure which is generated in the machine and reaches the tourniquet cuff via a tube. The amount of pressure and tourniquet time can be controlled by the machine. The display screen of the machine shows the tourniquet pressure and tourniquet time set for a particular operation.

Common Complications of Tourniquet

- Nerve paralysis
- Vessel injury
- Muscle injury
- Pulmonary embolism

The dangerous complication of a tourniquet is total ischaemia of the limb leading to tissue necrosis. If it is left for long hours, the viability of the distal limb will be lost and amputation may be the ultimate fate.

Tourniquet Time and Pressure

- There are no strict guidelines about safe tourniquet time and pressure. But most of the authors prefer 90 min with 250 mm Hg pressure for the upper limb and 120 min with 300 mm Hg pressure for the lower limb as safe tourniquet time and pressure, respectively.
- While using Esmarch's bandage as a tourniquet, the pressure is applied manually just to occlude the vessels but cannot be measured. If longer time is required, tourniquet should be released for 5 minutes and reapplied.

C-ARM IMAGE INTENSIFIER

- C-Arm image intensifier is a modified medical imaging device. It has two main parts: X-ray source and an X-ray detector. These two parts are connected by a C shaped metal arm which can move in multiple directions. That is why this machine is popularly known as C-Arm machine.
- The machine is also connected with a TV monitor to show the X-ray photograph of the different parts of the body of the patient. The best image is seen when the object is radio-opaque. The whole machine is mounted on wheels and can be moved from one place to another place (Fig. 39.6).

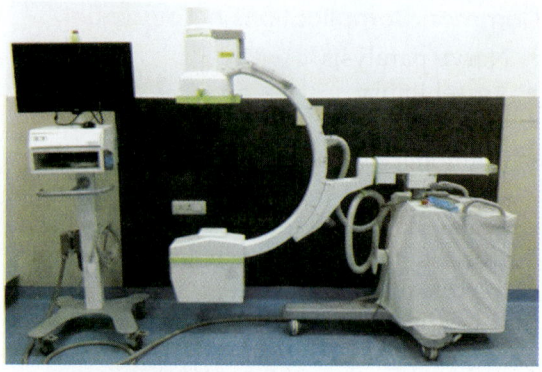

Fig. 39.6: C-Arm

Uses of the Machine

- In orthopaedic operations, to see the bones of the patients especially in fracture reduction and fixation with implants like nails, K-wires, plate, and screws.
- To see any metallic foreign body in the patient's body.
- To see the position of the catheter in cardiac surgery like pace making, angioplasty, etc.
- It is also used in other surgery to see the position of the organ and instruments.

Maintenance of the Machine

- Should remain fully covered by a plastic or cotton sheet when not in use.
- During surgery, the C-Arm, X-ray source and detector units are covered by a sterile plastic cover both for sterility and to avoid spillage of blood and other fluid on the machine parts.
- After surgery, the machine should be cleaned properly with a towel so that no blood or any other materials can adhere to any part of the machine which may cause rust formation.
- The wheels and other joints should be lubricated with machine oil as suggested by the manufacturing company.
- All measures are to be taken so that the machine is not exposed to dust and fumes like formalin or other chemicals. That can damage the software and finer electronic parts of the machine.

Special Precaution

- As it is a modified X-ray machine, there is a chance of radiation exposure. It has a cumulative effect on the body and the amount of exposure can be measured by thermoluminescent dosimeter (TLD).
- All persons present in the operation room must use a lead apron and TLD. Ideally one should use thyroid guard and special goggles to protect the eyes.
- It is also advised to protect the patient's body except the parts to be operated. This is more important in the case of a pregnant lady.

ENDOSCOPES

This is a long thin flexible or rigid tube with light and camera at the end and enters into the body through natural orifices of the body or through an incision over skin to visualize the interior and tissue spaces for diagnostic and treatment purposes. The scopes have an extra channel for operating instruments like electrosurgery probe and grasping or crushing forceps. The channels can also be used for suction and delivering gas and fluid into the abdomen. This scope has the facility to pass a sampling catheter for diagnostic purposes. Two types of endoscope are available: Rigid type and flexible type (Fig. 39.7).

Parts of Rigid Endoscope

- A metallic telescopic tube having no bending capacity when inserted into the body.
- Series of glass rod lenses designed to view objects at different angles.
- Eyepiece
- Light system
- Working channel through which instruments can be passed in some scopes
- Video monitor

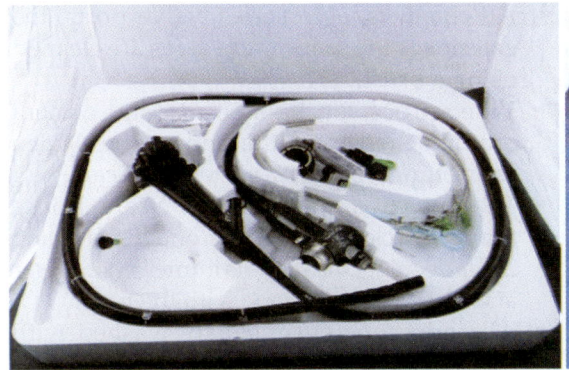 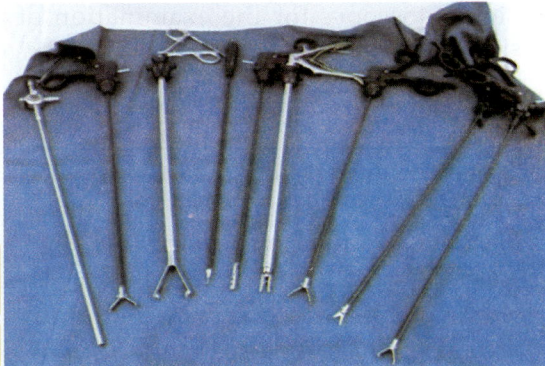

Fig. 39.7: Endoscope

Parts of Flexible Endoscope

- A thin long flexible insertion tube
- Lens system
- Illumination system
- Eyepiece
- Bending section at the distal tip of the insertion tube
- Control system
- Monitor to see the image and video

The endoscope has different names used in different locations and purposes as follows:

- Gastroscope *to visualize the interior of the stomach.*
- *Duodenoscope* to visualizes the interior of the duodenum.
- *Colonoscope* to visualize the interior of the colon.
- *Sigmoidoscope* to visualize the interior of the sigmoid colon.
- *Enteroscope* to visualize the interior of the intestine.
- *Bronchoscope* to visualize the interior of trachea and bronchus.
- *Laryngoscope* to visualize the interior of the larynx.
- *Cystoscope* to visualize the interior of the urinary bladder.

- *Ureteroscope* to visualize the interior of the ureter.
- *Hysteroscope* to visualize the interior of the uterus.
- *Colposcope* to visualize the interior of the vagina and opening of the cervix.
- *Arthroscope* to visualize the interior of the joint.
- *Neuroendoscope* to visualize the interior of the brain.
- *Thoracoscope* to visualize the interior of the chest.

Uses

- Laparoscopic biopsy from liver, pancreas, kidney, prostate, lymph node, small intestine.
- Examination of thorax and biopsy from pleura and lungs.
- Exploration of joint and arthroscopic surgery like cruciate ligament reconstruction.
- Endoscopic spine surgery like the removal of the intervertebral disc.
- Endoscopic ENT surgery (rhinoscopy) like removal of nasal polyp and biopsy from the maxillary sinus.
- Colposcopy surgery like cervical or vaginal wall biopsy.
- Gastroscopes used to see the stomach pathology.

- Sigmoidoscopes for the examination of sigmoid colon and biopsy.

Cleaning and Maintenance of Endoscope

- Immediately after use, the scope should be cleaned manually to remove the debris and dipped in enzymatic cleaning solution (instructed by the manufacturing company).
- After completion of the procedure, air or water valves are depressed and by regulating valve action mechanical cleaning of the channels is done by air and water.
- Sucking air and cleaning solution alternately by the tip of the scope internal lumens are made free from debris.

- All channels, accessories, valve ports, the exterior of the scope and valves are cleaned using a brush.
- Video processor, light source and camera are detached from the endoscope. Video connecting port is protected by a cap.
- The detached endoscope is cleaned once again with cleaning solution and disinfectant.
- After cleaning, the scope is immersed in water and the leak test is done with the tester.
- All endoscope channels are washed with the alcohol-water mixture, which is usually approximately 70–80 % alcohol. The alcohol helps to dry.
- The brush is checked whether it is frayed or damaged.

CHAPTER 40

Common Surgical Instruments

In the operation theatre, there are two types of surgical instruments. Some are general instruments required for every surgery and some are for specific surgical procedures.

Common surgical instruments are as follows:

- Artery forceps
- Dissecting forceps
- Towel clip
- Scissors
- Needle holder
- Scalpels
- Allis tissue forceps
- Sponge holding forceps
- Cheatle's forceps
- Kocher's forceps
- Sinus forceps
- Needles
- Scoop/curette
- Retractors

ARTERY FORCEPS

Artery forceps, also known as hemostatic forceps, are essential instruments in all surgical procedures to control bleeding.

Features

- Two ring handles
- Two long shanks
- Two locking ratchets
- Two serrated jaws
- Boxlock

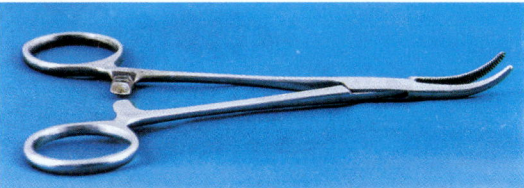

Fig. 40.1: Curved artery forceps

Types (Depending on its Size)

- **Large:** To catch large object (straight or curved; Fig. 40.1)
- **Medium** (straight or curved)
- **Small:** Also called mosquito forceps (straight or curved)

Uses

- To catch bleeding vessels
- To catch delicate soft tissue like peritoneum and pleura

DISSECTING FORCEPS

Dissecting forceps, also known as thumb forceps, are commonly used instruments for all surgical procedures to hold soft tissues including skin.

Features

It consists of two serrated wings connected at one end.

Types (Fig. 40.2)

- **Toothed dissecting forceps:** The tips of the wings have the tooth.
- **Non-toothed dissecting forceps:** The tips of the wings are plain

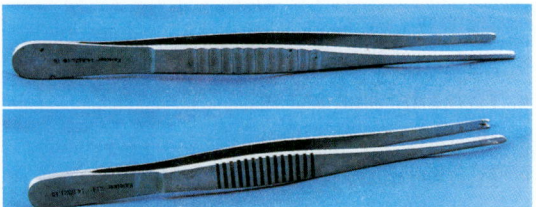

Fig. 40.2: Toothed and non-toothed thumb forceps

Uses

- To hold tough tissue of the body like skin, deep fascia, muscle, capsule, ligament and foreign body with toothed forceps.
- To hold delicate structures like nerve, peritoneum, and synovium.

TOWEL CLIP

It is an instrument used to secure drape and towels in an operative field. Different types of towel clips are available for different functions (Fig. 40.3).

Features of Typical Towel Clip

It consists of:
- Two ring handles
- Two long shanks
- Two locking ratchets
- Two pointed curved tips of the blades

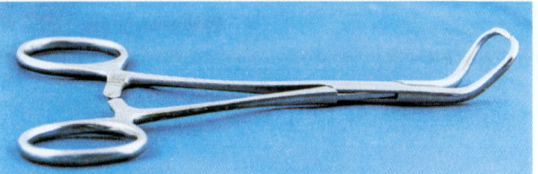

Fig. 40.3: Towel clip

Uses

- To fix the drapes with the body of the patient.
- To fix the diathermy cord or suction tube or any other similar items with the drapes near the operative field.
- To hold a small piece of bone or tough soft tissue.

SCISSORS

It is a cutting instrument used in the operative procedure (Fig. 40.4).

Features

- Two ring handles
- Two cutting blades /serrated jaws
- Two shafts/shanks
- Box lock (joint)

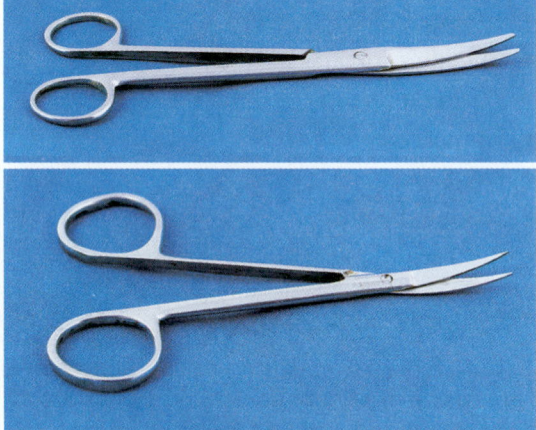

Fig. 40.4: Small and large scissors

Types

- Scissors with a long straight and curved blades.
- Scissors with short straight and curved blades.
- Scissors with short curved/straight and blunt/sharp-tipped blades.
- Scissors with specially designed short straight/curved blades.
- Specially designed stitch cutting scissors with curved small serrated blades.
- Heavy-duty scissors

Uses

- Straight long scissors to cut superficial tough structures.
- Curved long scissors to cut tough structures at a deeper plane.
- Straight short scissors to cut small delicate tissues in the surface.
- Curved short scissors to cut small delicate tissues in a deeper plane.
- Curved or straight scissors with blunt-tipped blades to dissect vessels and nerves.
- Scissors with small curved serrated blades to cut stitches.
- Heavy-duty scissors to cut gauze, bandage and draping materials.

NEEDLE HOLDERS

It is an instrument to hold needles of different sizes (Fig. 40.5).

Features

- Two ring handles
- Two short serrated jaws
- Two shafts/shanks
- Two locking ratchets
- Box lock (joint)

Types

- Long
- Medium
- Short

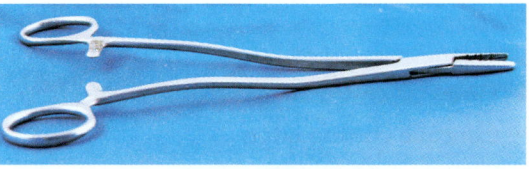

Fig. 40.5: Needle holder

- Curved
- Straight
- Angled

Uses

To grasp needles of different sizes for suturing tough to delicate tissue like skin and cornea, respectively.

SCALPEL

It is a cutting instrument with a reusable handle and a disposable blade.

Features of Handle (Fig. 40.6)

- Metallic handle
- Grooved narrow end to accommodate disposable blades of different series.
- Embossed with a number (4, 3 and 7 most commonly used)

Features of Blade

- Sharp cutting edge
- Straight or curved in shape
- A different shape for a different surgical procedure

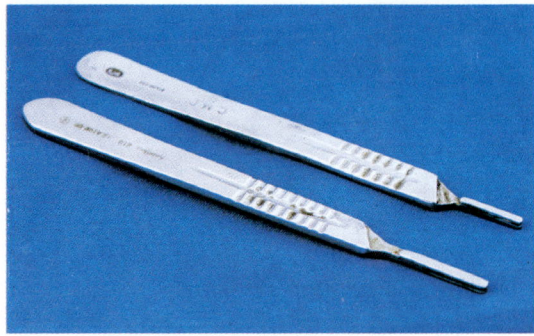

Fig. 40.6: Scalpel handle

Types

- Small
- Large
- Concave cutting edge
- Convex cutting edge
- Straight cutting edge

Uses

- To incise soft tissue like skin, fascia, membrane, muscle, tendon, capsule, ligament, etc.
- To incise an abscess cavity

ALLIS FORCEPS

It is a grasping and holding instrument.

Features

- Two ring handles
- Two jaws
- Multiple teeth at the tip of the jaws in row
- Two shafts
- Two locking ratchets
- Box lock (joint)

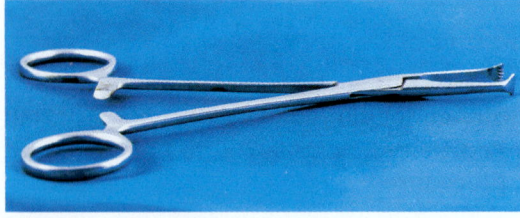

Fig. 40.7: Allis forceps

Types

- Long
- Short
- Curved sometimes

Uses

- To grasp the tough structure
- To hold soft tissue for dissection

SPONGE-HOLDING FORCEPS

It is a holding instrument basically designed to hold a sponge or swab about 9 inches in length.

Features

- Two ring handles
- Two jaws
- Two shafts
- Two locking ratchets
- Box lock (joint)

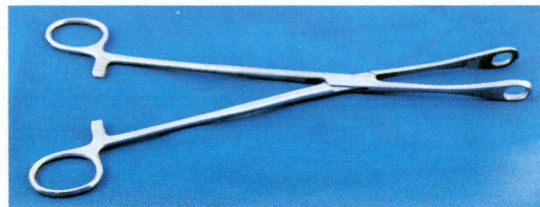

Fig. 40.8: Sponge-holding forceps

Types

- Straight
- Curved

Uses

- To hold sponge for cleaning/painting the skin before surgery
- To toilet the abdominal cavity after surgery
- To hold fundus of the gallbladder

CHEATLE'S FORCEPS

It is a heavy metallic forceps designed to hold and move sterilized instruments and materials from one place to another.

The instrument is kept in a wide mouth jar filled with an antiseptic lotion. One must be careful that the tip of the forceps does not touch unsterile area (Fig. 40.9).

Features

- Two ring handles
- Two angled shafts

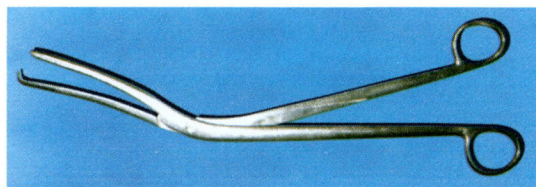

Fig. 40.9: Cheatle's forceps

- Two serrated jaws
- No locking device
- Joint in midshaft region

Uses

To hold sterile instruments or drape or any other item from a sterile drum usually.

KOCHER'S HAEMOSTATIC FORCEPS

This forceps has almost similar features of haemostatic forceps or artery forceps (Fig. 40.10).

Features

- Two ring handles
- Two long shanks
- Two locking ratchets
- Two serrated jaws
- Box lock
- Tip of the jaws are toothed (Fig. 40.10)

Types

- Straight and curved
- Long and short

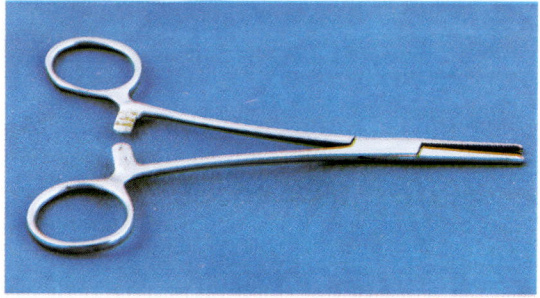

Fig: 40.10: Kocher's haemostatic forceps

Uses

- To catch bleeding vessels in tough tissues (like palm, sole of the foot)
- To hold any tough structure firmly during surgical dissection.

SINUS FORCEPS

It has almost all the features of the grasping instrument except the lock mechanism. The jaws are long and serrated.

It is used to explore any sinus tract or abscess cavity. As there is no lock, it cannot catch any important soft tissue during its manoeuvre.

SCOOP/CURETTE

It is a spoon-shaped instrument with a handle of various sizes. The margin of the spoon is sharp. It is used to scrape abnormal or normal tissue during debridement, biopsy or removal of a foreign body (Fig. 40.11).

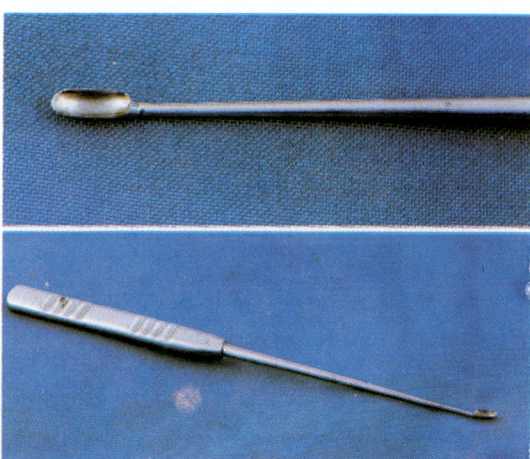

Fig: 40.11: Curette

SURGICAL NEEDLE

It is a metallic device used to suture a surgical or non-surgical wound. It works when an attached thread passes through margins of the wound and the thread is tightened with the help of a needle holder. The needles are available in different shapes and sizes for suturing different types of tissues (Fig. 40.12).

Parts of the Needle

- An eye for attachment of thread
- Body
- Tip

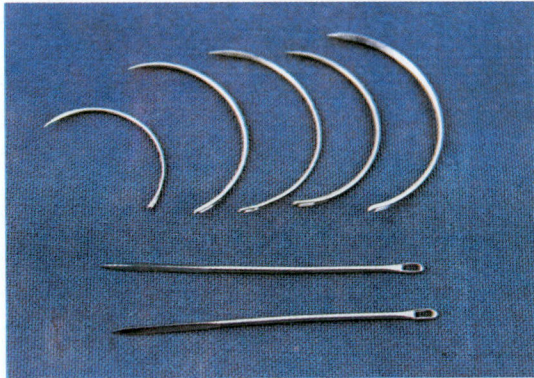

Fig. 40.12: Surgical needle

Types

- Straight
- Curved (the curvature may be 1/4, 3/8, 1/2, or 5/8 circle and it is easy to manoeuvre the needle in a small space with a more curved needle)
- Cutting with sharp edges at the tip
- Round bodied needle which can pass through delicate soft tissue like peritoneum.
- Atraumatic needle: In this needle, thread blends with the closed eye without increasing its diameter so as to pass through the tissue with less damage.

Uses

- Straight needles are used for suturing skin usually.
- Curved cutting needles are used for suturing tough tissues like skin, capsule, and fascia.
- The curved round-bodied needle is used for repair of muscle and other soft tissues.

- The very small curved needle is used for suturing delicate tissues like nerve and cornea or similar structures.

RETRACTOR

It is a basic instrument used to separate the margins of a surgical incision or wound. During surgical dissection, the organs and other tissues are separated for better visibility of the desired site. Depending upon the surgical site and procedure, the retractors are designed in various shapes and sizes. Commonly Langenbeck 'L' shaped or Deaver 'C' shaped retractors are used in most of the general and abdominal surgeries. The retractors may be manual or self-retaining (Fig. 40.13).

Parts of a Typical Retractor

- Handle for holding with the hands
- One blade or hook of different shape and sizes at one end of the shaft

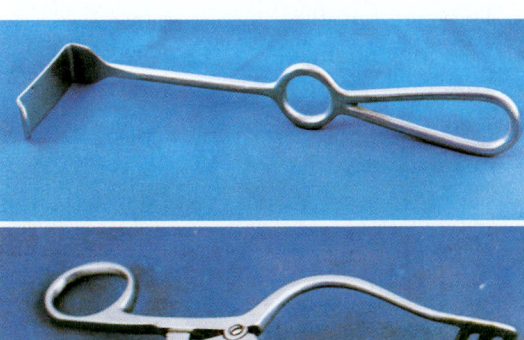

Fig. 40.13: Langenbeck and self-retaining retractors

Uses

- It is a basic instrument and required for every surgery for retraction of wound margins
- This is one of the essential items like artery or thumb forceps in any instrument trolley.

CHAPTER 41

Orthopaedic, Gynaecological and Obstetric, Ophthalmic, Otolaryngologic, Endoscopic, Cardiothoracic and Neurosurgical Instruments

ORTHOPAEDIC INSTRUMENTS

Common Instruments

- Periosteal elevator (different sizes) to remove periosteum from the bone surface with muscle or other soft tissue.
- Osteotome (straight, curved and different sizes) for cutting bone.
- Chisel (sloping edge, straight, curved and different sizes) for making a window in a bone.
- Gouge (straight, curved and different sizes) for making a window in the bone.
- Bone cutting forceps (straight, curved and different sizes) for cutting small bones or a piece of bone.
- Bone nibbler (straight, curved and different sizes) for nibbling a bone or tough tissue attached with the bone.
- Bone cutting saw (different sizes) for cutting bone end (amputation).
- Gigli saw (handle with wire) for cutting bone where working space is limited.
- Bone file or rasp for smoothening of rough bone ends (usually after amputation surgery).
- Mallet or hammer to strike osteotome, chisel, gouge, and intramedullary nail.
- Bone awl for making a hole in the bone.

- Bradol (has one eye) for making a hole in the bone.
- Bone lever (different shapes and sizes) for lifting the bone from its bed and retraction of soft tissue from the bone surface.
- Hohmann retractor (different sizes) for retracting soft tissue from the bone.
- Bone hook for manipulating the fragment from its bed.
- Bone-holding forceps (different configurations) for holding and manipulating bone fragments.
- Sequestrum forceps (locking device) for holding.
- Hand drill for drilling bone.
- Screw driver for inserting a screw into the bone.
- Drill bit (different diameters) for making a hole in the bone for insertion of a screw
- Bone tap (different diameters) for making a thread in the bone hole for easy insertion of a screw.
- Bone punch to strike on projected bones and metallic substance to be in the desired place.
- K-wire (different diameters) for provisional or definitive fixation of small bone fragments.

- Stainless steel wire (different gauze) commonly used for fixation of fracture fragments of patella, olecranon as tension band wiring.
- Steinmann pin used for skeletal traction mainly.
- Intramedullary K-nail (assorted sizes and diameter) for fixation of long bone fracture (in femur, tibia, and humerus).
- Intramedullary interlocking nail (assorted sizes and diameter) for fixation of long bone fracture (in femur, tibia, and humerus) has proximal and distal holes for screw fixation to prevent rotation at the fracture site.
- Intramedullary Ender's flexible nail (assorted sizes and diameter) for fixation of long bone fracture (in femur, tibia, and humerus)
- Rash rod (assorted sizes and diameter) for fixation of long bone fracture. It is round-shaped and prevents rotation when the hook, in the end, is buried into the bone.
- Square nail (assorted sizes and diameter) for fixation of long bone fracture. It is a flexible nail and its square shape prevents rotation when inserted into the medullary canal.
- **Screw:** It is an important basic implant for fixation of fracture fragments or a plate with the bone. It is also used to prevent rotation when placed in locking holes of intramedullary nails. Its head, shaft, and tip have different designs to serve different functions and available in assorted size and diameter.
- **Plate:** It has a different shape, size, and design used for fixation of bone fragments (available for use in different locations).

Commonly used plates are:

- Plate without compression device
- Plate with compression device (having oval plate holes) called dynamic compression plate (DCP). Narrow DCP is used for radius, ulna, fibula and broad DCP for femur, tibia, and humerus.
- Mini-fragment plate is a very small plate in length, thickness and breadth used for fixation of fractures of small bones of hand and foot.
- The contoured plate is designed for use in proximal and distal long bones like femur, tibia, and humerus.
- The locking plate has threads in holes for screw fixation.
- Low contact dynamic compression plate (LCDCP).
- Buttress plate
- Semitubular plate

- **Dynamic hip screw:** Fixation device in trochanteric fracture of the femur.
- **Prosthesis:** It is a device which replaces one or both parts of a joint.
  - *Thompson prosthesis/Austin Moore's prosthesis:* Replaces hip joint (head and neck of femur in fracture neck of femur in an elderly patient).
  - *Knee prosthesis:* Replaces a part or whole of the knee joint.
  - *Elbow prosthesis:* Replaces elbow joint.
  - *Shoulder prosthesis:* Replaces shoulder joint.
  - *Ankle prosthesis:* Replaces ankle joint.
  - *Radial head prosthesis:* Replaces head of the radius

Common orthopaedic instruments are shown in Figs 41.1 and 41.2.

Arthroscope

This is a machine by which a surgeon can visualize the internal structures of a joint. Common joints where it is used are knee, shoulder, hip, elbow, ankle, and wrist. The arthroscope helps to diagnose and treat many joint diseases and injuries.

Parts of Arthroscope Machine

- Scope—a rigid tube with a lens system entering the joint
- Optical fibre—surrounding the lens which transmits light to the joint from the source

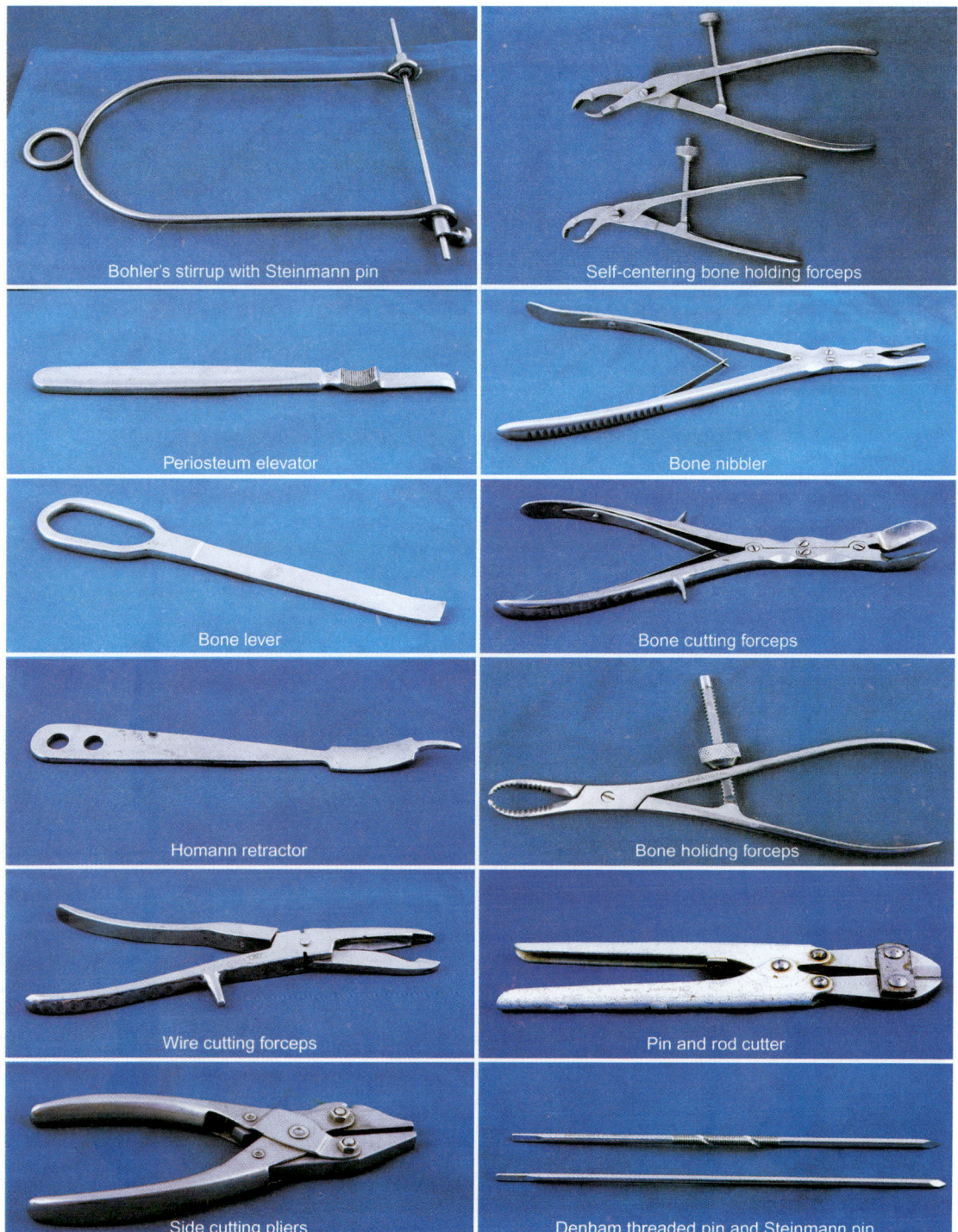

Fig. 41.1: Common orthopaedic instruments

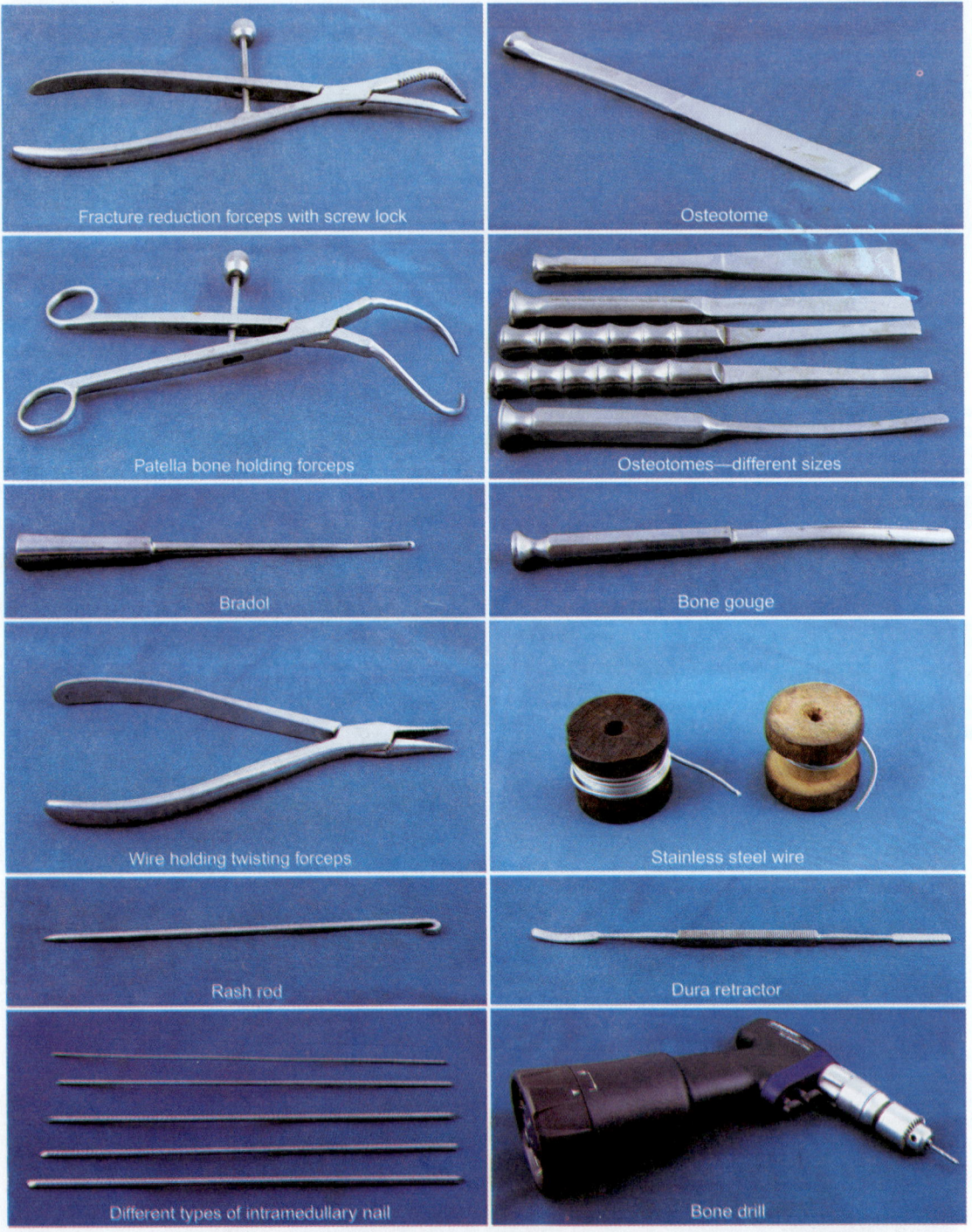

Fracture reduction forceps with screw lock

Osteotome

Patella bone holding forceps

Osteotomes—different sizes

Bradol

Bone gouge

Wire holding twisting forceps

Stainless steel wire

Rash rod

Dura retractor

Different types of intramedullary nail

Bone drill

Fig. 41.2: Common orthopaedic instruments and implants

- Eyepiece—fitted with a camera which captures a photograph of internal structures of joint.
- Light source—which transmits light to the scope through a cable.
- Video monitor—showing the camera pictures of the joint on the screen.

Arthroscopic system means:

- Arthroscope
- Light source
- Light cable
- Camera system
- Video recorder monitor
- Arthroscopic instruments
- Irrigation system
- Suction pump
- Special hand instruments

COMMON INSTRUMENTS FOR GYNAECOLOGICAL AND OBSTETRICAL OPERATION

- Sims vaginal speculum—to inspect the vagina and cervix.
- Cusco's vaginal speculum—to inspect the vagina and cervix.
- Cervical dilator (Hegar's)—to dilate the opening of the cervix for D&C and D&E operations.
- Vulsellum forceps—to hold the lip of cervix
- Ovum forceps—to remove placental fragments and products of conception in incomplete or inevitable abortion from the uterine cavity.
- Sim's uterine sound—to measure the length and direction of the cervix and uterus.
- Uterine curette (double-ended)—for removing tissues from the inner lining of the uterus.
- Myomectomy clamp (Bonney)—used to remove the uterine fibroid.
- Cervical biopsy forceps—used to take a biopsy from the cervix.
- Punch biopsy forceps—used to take a small amount of tissue from a selected area of the cervix.

- Shirodkar's uterus holding forceps—used to hold the uterus in operations like salpingectomy and cervical amputation.
- Endometrial biopsy curette-for sampling endometrial lining.
- Episiotomy scissors, non-ratcheted, blunt-angled scissors—to perform episiotomy during labour and delivery.
- Bladder sound—to locate any stone in the bladder.
- Anterior vaginal wall retractor placed on the posterior wall and to examine the anterior wall of the vagina to check any inflammatory lesions of the pelvis.
- Polypus forceps—used to remove a polyp from the uterus.
- Uterine dressing forceps multifunctional instrument for packing uterine cavity or removal of tissues after the D&C procedure.
- Cranioclast—to crush and then extract the skull of a fetus to facilitate delivery in obstructed labour.
- Green Armytage uterine forceps—used to grasp and clamp tissues in the uterus.
- Flushing curette (blunt type)—used to collect a sample from uterus or rectum.
- Endometrial biopsy curette—used to collect endometrial tissue from the uterus.
- Auvard weighted speculum is a single end vaginal speculum. Used in vaginal hysterectomy.
- Hawkins Ambler's uterine dilators—single-ended uterine dilators of various widths.
- Obstetrical forceps for delivery of fetal head having two large jaws for holding used in vaginal delivery of the baby.

COMMON INSTRUMENTS FOR ENT SURGERY

- Tonsil holding forceps look like sponge holding forceps. Used in tonsillectomy operation.
- Davis Boyle mouth gag—used in tonsillectomy and adenoidectomy operations.
- Tonsillar artery forceps (straight and curved)—used in tonsillectomy operation.

- Tonsillar scissor—used in tonsillectomy operation.
- Tonsil dissector—used in tonsillectomy operation.
- Tonsil dissector and retractor combined. Used in tonsillectomy operation.
- The tonsillar snare is used in tonsillectomy operations.
- Adenoid curette used in adenoidectomy.
- The head mirror is used in the ENT examination.
- The aural speculum is used in the examination of the ear.
- Siegle speculum (pneumatic speculum)— used in the examination of the ear.
- Nasal speculum (long-bladed)—used in SMR and turbinectomy.
- Nasal speculum (short-bladed)—used in the examination of the nose (anterior rhinoscopy).
- Metallic tongue depressor straight and curved used in the examination of the oral cavity and oropharynx.
- Wooden tongue depressor used in the examination of the oral cavity and oropharynx.
- The laryngeal mirror is used in the examination of the larynx (indirect laryngoscopy).
- The post-nasal mirror used in the examination of the posterior part of the nasal cavity and nasopharynx (posterior rhinoscopy).
- Dressing forceps—used for dressing of the ear or nose.
- Probe (cotton applicator)—used for cleaning the ear canal.
- Tuning fork. Diagnostic instrument.
- Self-retaining nasal speculum—used for SMR and septoplasty operations.
- Luc's forceps—used for SMR and turbinectomy.
- Septal dissector—used for SMR and septoplasty operations.
- A nasal snare—used for polypectomy operation.
- Chisel—used for SMR and Caldwell-Luc operations.

- Antral burr—used for intranasal inferior antrostomy.
- Ethmoid curette—used in intranasal ethmoidectomy operation.
- Periosteal elevator—used in mastoidectomy and Caldwell-Luc operations.
- Swivel knife—used in SMR and septoplasty operations.
- Metallic sucker (suction tip)—used in SMR, turbinectomy and other nasal operations.
- Walsham's forceps—used in the reduction of fractured nasal bones.
- Anterior nasal pack—used in the management of anterior epistaxis.
- Posterior nasal pack—used in the management of posterior epistaxis.
- Myringotomy knife—used for myringotomy operation.
- Mastoid curette—used in mastoidectomy operation.
- Gland forceps—used in thyroidectomy and submandibular sialadenectomy.
- Alice forceps—used in tracheostomy and neck operations.
- Tracheal dilator—used in tracheostomy operation.
- Tracheostomy tube (single lumen, silicon, cuffed)—used in tracheostomy operation.

Common ENT instruments are shown in Fig. 41.3.

Laser Instrument

Laser surgery is a surgical procedure where special light beams are used instead of surgical instruments while performing the surgeries. Full form of 'LASER' is "light amplification by stimulated emission of radiation". Laser device produces light which has no existence in nature. It has three characteristics:

- One colour or wavelength (so-called monochromatic).
- Wavelengths are in phases (called coherent).
- Light beams are very narrow and concentrated on one point (called collimated).

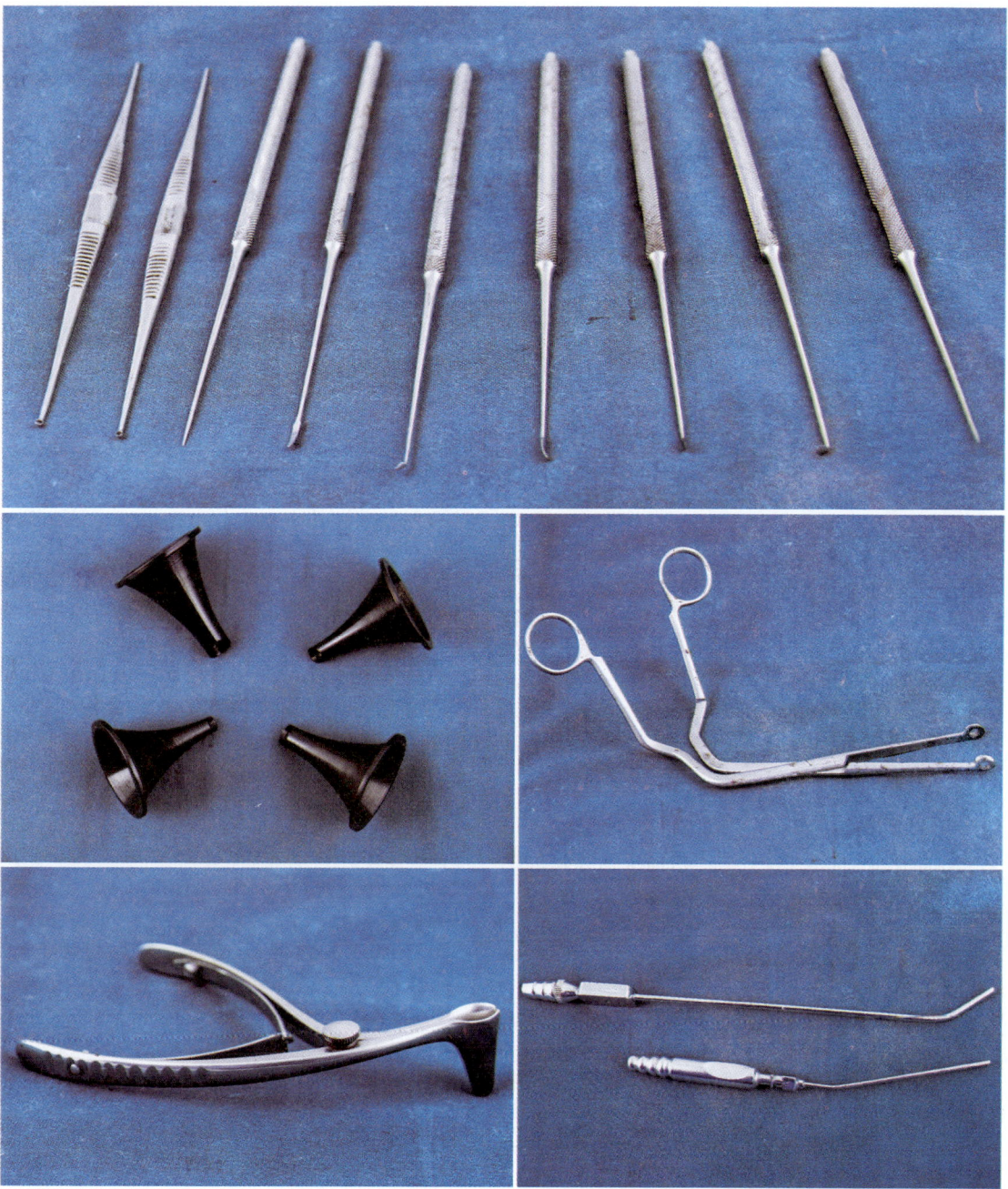

Fig. 41.3: Common ENT instruments

Basically, the uses of lasers in soft tissue surgery are to cut, ablate, vapourize, and coagulate. With this principle, laser is used in many ophthalmic, ENT, dental, maxillo-facial, tumour neurosurgery and other surgeries nowadays.

The laser is constructed from three principal components:

- Lasing medium
- External energy source
- Optical resonator

Uses of Laser

- Dermatology and plastic surgery—to remove unwanted scar, vascular and pigmented lesion.
- Eye surgery—to correct the refractive error and to remove corneal opacity.
- Vascular surgery—to remove atheroma in the artery and laser-assisted angioplasty.
- Foot and ankle surgery—to remove a tumour from talus and calcaneum and to treat ingrowing nail.
- Gastrointestinal surgery—to treat oesophageal varices and duodenal ulcers (photoablation), haemorrhoids, colorectal and liver cancer.
- Spine surgery such as discectomy operation
- Used in dental, gynecological, urogenital, thoracic, neurosurgery, otolaryngological surgeries.

COMMON INSTRUMENTS FOR OPHTHALMIC SURGERY

- Speculum used for keeping the eye open during operation.
- Guarded eye speculum (left and right) keeps eyelashes away from the operative field.
- Universal eye speculum can be used in both eyes for keeping the eye open during operation. This is used in a squint, pterygium, foreign body removal from cornea operations.
- Needle holders (light weight)—for holding needles.
- Arruga's needle holder with a catch (lock) for heavy-duty.
- Barraquer's needle holder without a catch for light duty.

- Artery forceps (haemostat)—to catch blood vessels.
- Plain dissecting forceps—to hold soft tissues without damage.
- Colibri forceps—for holding corneal flaps.
- Iris forceps to hold iris.
- Superior rectus holding forceps—to hold rectus muscle.
- Capsulotomy forceps—used in cataract surgery.
- McPherson's forceps—for holding parts of the lens.
- Chalazion forceps (clamp)—used in chalazion surgery.
- Epilation forceps (Cilia forceps)—for removing eyelashes.
- Diamond knife—used for microincision on the cornea.
- Nettleship's punctum dilator—used for dilating the lacrimal punctum.
- Wire Vectis—for lens extraction
- Lacrimal cannula—for introducing drugs and fluids into the nasolacrimal duct.
- Evisceration spoon or scoop—for removing contents of the eyeball during evisceration.
- Tookes' knife has semi-circular cutting edge used in cataract operation and also for splitting layers of the sclera.
- Elliot's trephine with handle—for corneal surgery.
- Rougine—for dissection of the lacrimal duct
- Strabismus hook, muscle hook or squint hook—used for squint surgery.
- Elsching's intracapsular forceps
- Keratome both straight and angle bladed knife—used for incising cornea.
- Disc holding forceps.
- Lens expressor—used in cataract surgery
- Lens spatula—used in cataract surgery.
- Castroviejo corneal spring scissors has double spring used in operations of cornea and iris.

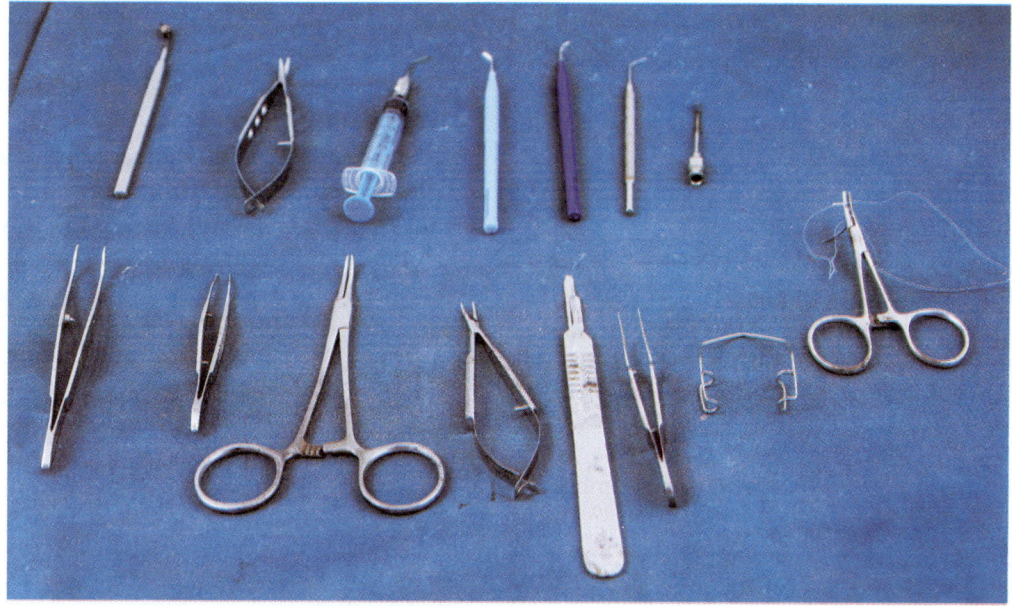

Fig. 41.4: Common ophthalmic surgical instruments

- Conjunctiva forceps—used to hold conjunctival and episcleral tissues together and also to catch episcleral bleeding vessels.
- Ziegler's knife needle—for disrupting lens materials.
- Vectis cannula—for removal and irrigation of nucleus.
- Punctum dilator—used for dilatation of lacrimal punctum.
- Cat's paw retractor—used to retract delicate structures.

Common ophthalmic surgical instruments are shown in Fig. 41.4.

COMMON INSTRUMENTS FOR NEUROSURGERY

- Gigli saw with hook handle—used for cutting skull bone
- Skull cutting forceps—used in craniotomy operation and essential instrument for all brain surgery almost.
- Trephine—used for all surgeries through the skull for perforation in the bone.
- Dural hook—used to retract, lift and tough outer layer of the brain.

- Dura retractor—to retract nerve roots and dural sac.
- Penfield dissector double-ended with a broad curved dissector and a rounded spoon.
- Pituitary forceps have cup-shaped jaws used in the pituitary operation.
- Adson's periosteal elevator—to elevate muscle and periosteum from the bone.
- Ventricular drainage cannula—a plastic tube placed in the ventricle of the brain to drain cerebrospinal fluid in hydrocephalus.
- Brain suction tube has a special design that prevents clogging.
- Hudson's brace with burs and drills—used in perforation of the skull bone.

Operating Microscope

It is an optical microscope used in many surgical specialties. By this device, the surgeon can visualize the illuminated and magnified image of very small structures in the operative field.

Components of Microscope

- Binocular head with an attached telescope having adjustable eyepieces
- Objective lens
- Prism
- Magnification changer
- Illuminator
- Floor stand with attached suspension arm
- Optical system attached with the suspension arm
- Foot pedal connected to the floor stand to control focus, zoom, and illumination

Uses

- Ophthalmic surgery (posterior chamber)
- Otolaryngologic surgery
- Neurosurgery
- Plastic surgery

Maintenance of Equipment

- The microscope should be kept in a dry cool and well-ventilated place to avoid the growth of fungus in the lens.
- Weekly cleaning of the optics as instructed by the manufacturing company.
- Foot pedal to cover in a plastic bag to avoid damage by blood, body fluid and water.
- To use voltage stabilizer with the microscope to avoid fluctuation of voltage which might destroy the bulbs of the device.
- To avoid kinking and bending of the fiberoptic cables.
- Not to move the microscope when the bulbs are hot. The hot filaments may be damaged by vibrations.
- Brake oil should be used every 6 months in the wheels.
- The whole unit should be covered by the vinyl cover to protect the electronic gadgets of the unit from dust particles.

COMMON INSTRUMENTS FOR PLASTIC SURGERY

- Skin grafting knife—for harvesting skin from the donor site.

- Angular scissors are used in a few reconstructive dental and ophthalmic surgeries.
- Adson's brown forceps—for holding and manipulating delicate tissues.
- Denis Brown cleft palate raspatory—used in hare lip and cleft palate surgery.
- Kilner scissors curved and scissors used to cut delicate structures.
- Joseph rasp is a tool for contouring nasal reconstructive surgeries.
- Nasal chisel—used for rhinoplasty.
- Iris scissors having short blades—used in cutting delicate structures.

COMMON INSTRUMENTS FOR UROLOGICAL SURGERY

- Metal urethral catheter
- Bladder irrigation syringe—used for the irrigation of the bladder after any operation in the bladder.
- Toomey syringe—for bladder irrigation after TURP operation.
- Urethral dilator—commonly used in the stricture of the urethra.
- Millin's bladder neck dilator—used in bladder neck stricture.
- Cystolithotomy forceps—used to remove bladder stones.
- Trocar and cannula—used in different surgeries like suprapubic cystostomy.
- Morris kidney retractor—used in kidney surgery.
- Nephrolithotomy forceps—used to remove stones in the kidney usually through an incision in the skin.
- Boomerang needle holder has a spring mechanism in the handle for attachment of different types of needles.

COMMON INSTRUMENTS FOR CARDIOVASCULAR SURGERY

- Bulldog clamp is used to occlude arteries especially in surgery for coronary artery.

- Aortic cross-clamp—used to clamp aorta and to separate systemic circulation from the cardiac outflow.

- Aortic anastomosis clamps—special type of clamp to occlude the lumen of aorta in thoracic aortic surgery.

- Patent ductus arteriosus (PDA) clamp has special curvature which allows efficient bite over the aortic and pulmonary wall in PDA surgery.

- An embolectomy catheter is a long tube with an inflatable balloon at the tip used to remove emboli in the vessel.

- The cardiac catheter is a long tube introduced into the heart through vessels in different interventional procedures for heart and coronary artery disease.

- Cardiac retractor—used in coronary bypass operation.

- Empyema trochar and cannula—to drain any fluid in the thoracic cavity.

- Lung holding forceps are large light-weight grasping forceps to handle weak slippery organs like stomach and lungs.

Common instruments for cardiovascular surgery are shown in Fig. 41.5.

Special Equipment in Cardiothoracic Surgery

Heart-Lung Machine

It is a device that temporarily takes the function of lungs and heart. It is also called a cardiac bypass pump or cardiopulmonary bypass machine. In some surgical procedures, the heart needs to be kept empty but during that period, the tissues of the body will require oxygen for their survival. The heart-lung machine provides oxygenated blood during that period. Venous blood of the body is drained through disposable plastic tube into the reservoir from where a roller pump moves the blood to the heat exchanger and oxygenator. Oxygenation of blood occurs in this

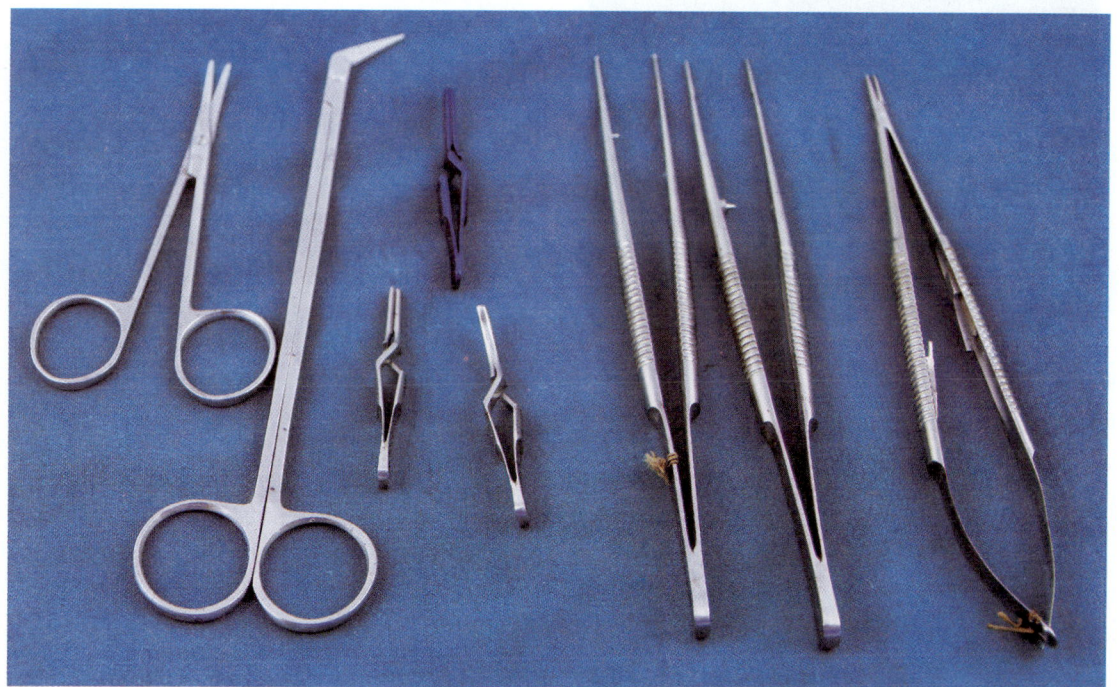

Fig. 41.5: Common instruments for cardiovascular surgeries

section and carbon dioxide is removed. Oxygenated blood is then delivered into the arterial system. Temporarily the bypass machine performs the functions of lungs and heart till the heart stars beating. The role of a person, called perfusionist, is very important who operates this heart-lung machine. He is to look after this artificial blood pump which propels oxygenated blood in general circulation with normal or near-normal concentration blood gases (Fig. 41.6).

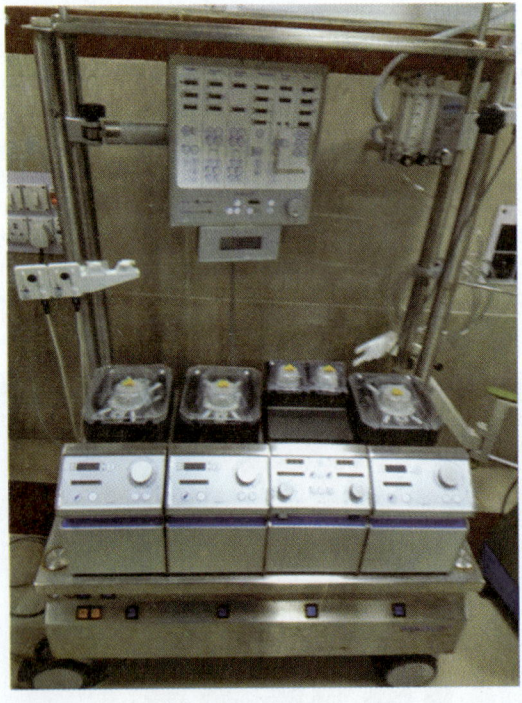

Fig. 41.6: Heart-lung machine

Components of machine

- **Pump:** There are two types of pump. Centrifugal pump produces pulse less blood flow and less destructive to blood elements. The roller pump compresses a segment of tubes for forwarding the flow of blood. It is pulsatile but there is a chance of hemolysis.
- The venous cannula (plastic bag and a place to add drugs, fluid, and blood)

- Arterial cannula
- Venous reservoir
- Disposable plastic tubing
- **Oxygenator:** Membranous oxygenator imitates normal lungs. Only oxygen and carbon dioxide can pass through the membrane. In bubble oxygenator, venous blood drains directly into a chamber where oxygen is infused through a diffusion plate which produces oxygen bubbles and surface of oxygen bubbles acts as a membrane for gaseous exchange.
- **Heat exchanger:** It regulates the temperature of the blood.
- **Filter and bubble traps:** Filtering the bubbles before entering into the arterial system.
- **Perfusion monitor and sensors:** Here bubbles can be detected and the concentration of gases can be measured along with the temperature of the blood.

Uses of heart-lung machine

- In most of the surgeries for congenital anomalies of the heart diseases like ventricular septal defect and atrial septal defect.
- In valve replacement surgery
- In ventricular aneurysm repair
- Carotid endarterectomy
- Transmyocardial laser revascularization
- In heart transplant surgery

CLEANING AND MAINTENANCE OF EQUIPMENT

Cleaning

The instruments used during a surgical procedure are soiled with blood, body fluids and tissue debris. These are reusable and cleaned after each surgery and kept ready for the next operation. The steps of cleaning are as follows:

- All soiled instruments are placed under running warm water for a few minutes and rinsed to remove blood clots and other materials. Then these are submerged in neutral pH detergent solution for more cleaning. Soft plastic brushes are used for cleaning manually. The hinges and locks of instruments are areas of hidden blood clots and tissue debris and that should be cleaned properly with a small brush. Delicate and sharp instruments should be handled carefully to avoid breakage loss of sharpness.

- The instruments can be cleaned by the ultrasonic method where instruments are submerged into the cleaning solution for about 5–10 minutes. Then it is again washed with water to remove the previous solution.

- After cleaning, the extra water is removed with the help of a soft towel and kept open in the air to make them completely dry.

- Dry instruments are then lubricated with surgical lubricants after which the instruments are either stored in the box in order or sent for autoclaving after proper wrapping for the next operation.

Checking and Maintenance

- While cleaning it is advised to check different parts of the instruments especially the hinges and locks.

- The tips or business parts of instruments like hemostat forceps, needle holding forceps, tooth forceps, Allis forceps, towel clip, and others are aligned perfectly when locked. Tightly aligned tips of hemostat and needle holders will not allow light to pass through the jaws. This is a simple test to check their functional status.

- The pointed tips of towel clip forceps should meet each other properly and can catch a piece of cloth firmly after locking.

- During cleaning, the functional status of all instruments is checked and defective instruments are identified and kept separately. The sharpness of the sharp instruments like scissors, knife, osteotome, and chisel are checked routinely.

- Any kind of visible stains on the surface or hinges are looked for and cleaned properly.

- It is important to note that the weight of heavy instruments might deform the delicate instruments when mixed together. Such items should be kept and handled separately to avoid damage.

- Suction tubes and other hollow and tubular instruments are inspected for the presence of blood clots or tissue fragments inside. These are washed placing under running tap water and soft non-metallic thin brushes are used for cleaning the tubes.

- While cleaning and checking sharp instruments and implants, one should be cautious about self-injury. Cleaning, rinsing, and checking of instruments are done in gloved hands only to avoid injury and contamination.

- The cleaning and maintenance of special instruments of different surgeries have been discussed in respective chapters.

CHAPTER 42

Anaesthetic Machine

The modern anaesthetic machine is a continuous flow type of machine. It receives medical gases under pressure, creates a gas mixture of the desired composition with known concentrations of inhalational agents and delivers fresh gas flow at a rate set by an anaesthesiologist.

Anaesthesia work station includes modern anaesthesia machine, circle breathing system and anaesthesia ventilator.

Anaesthesia machine consists of following functional anatomy sections.

- Gas supply system
- Anaesthesia vapourizers
- Anaesthesia breathing system
- Anaesthesia ventilator

GAS SUPPLY SYSTEM

High-Pressure System: Gas Cylinders

- Gas cylinders are made of molybdenum steel to withstand high pressure.
- Cylinders are available in different sizes (Table 42.1)
- 'E' size cylinders are used on the anaesthesia machine
- They are colour coded.
  - **Oxygen:** Black body white shoulder
  - **Nitrous oxide:** Blue
  - **Air:** Grey body white and black shoulder
- The upper part of the cylinder ends in a tapered screw called neck. This is threaded into the valve.

Table 42.1	Cylinder size and capacity					
Cylinder gas capacity	**Cylinder size**					
	C	**D**	**E**	**F**	**G**	**J**
Oxygen (L)	170	340	680	1360	3400	6800
N$_2$O (L)	450	900	1800	3600	9000	–
Air (L)	–	–	–	–	3200	6400

- The cylinder outlet valve contains a pin index system, which makes it impossible to connect the cylinder to the wrong yolk assembly.
- Yoke contains two metal pins and corresponding filling holes present on the cylinder valve.
- Marks engraved on the cylinder are:
  - Test pressure (cylinder tested at pressure by manufacturer)
  - Date of test performed
  - The chemical formula of the content of the cylinder
  - Tare weight (weight of the empty cylinder)
  - Serial number
  - Name of the owner
- The cylinder valve should be slightly opened and then closed before connecting to the anaesthesia machine. This is called cracking of the cylinder, which clears particles of dust and grease from the exit port.
- After connection to the anaesthesia machine, the cylinder valve is slowly opened 2.5 turns and check the pressure gauge for the amount of gas present in the cylinder.
- Most of the modern anaesthesia machines are connected to gas pipelines for continuous uninterrupted supply of gas. Cylinders attached to the machine are mostly kept as a reserve for emergency use.

Pressure Gauge

Pressure gauge measures the pressure of the cylinder or pipeline. It is Bourdon type tube pressure gauge.

Pressure Regulator

The preset pressure regulator reduces the pressure to 400 kPa. It converts variable high cylinder pressure to constant low operating pressure.

Intermediate Pressure Zone

The pressure of the intermediate zone is approximately 400 kPa. The intermediate zone consists of gas pipelines, oxygen flush valve, oxygen supply failure alarm, oxygen failure protection device or fail-safe valve.

Gas Pipelines

- The main source of medical gas in a large hospital is gas manifold. Oxygen can also be stored in a liquid oxygen tank.
- From central supply, medical gases are delivered to different sites in the hospital by pipelines.
- Oxygen, nitrous oxide, air and medical vacuum are commonly provided through the pipeline system.
- Outlets are identified by colour coding, gas name and shape. Flexible colour-coded pipelines run from anaesthesia machine to the outlet.
- Diameter index safety system (DISS) connectors are used to prevent cross-connection or misconnection. Once gas enters into anaesthesia machine through DISS connector. It cannot move in the reverse direction due to the one-way valve.

Oxygen Flush Valve

It provides manual delivery of 100% oxygen directly to the breathing system at 400 kPa pressure.

Oxygen Supply Failure Alarm

It activates, if oxygen supply pressure falls below 200 kPa. It is an audible signal. An alarm system does not base on the power supply or battery.

Oxygen Failure Protection Device or Fail-Safe Valve

If the pressure of oxygen drops at intermediate zone, the fail-safe valve shut off or proportionately decreases the flow of other gases.

Low-Pressure Section

It includes flow control valve, flow meter, anti-hypoxic system and common gas outlet.

Flow Control Valve

- A needle valve controls the flow of gases manually by turning a control knob in the clockwise or anti-clockwise direction.
- Control knob controls the forward or backward movements of the needle and thus changes the size of the passage and the amount of gases flow through it.
- Flow control knobs are labelled and colour coded.

Flowmeter

- Flowmeter measures the flow rate of a gas. They are individually calibrated for each gas.
- Rotameter is a type of flow meter, consists of transparent glass or plastic tube with a tapering cross-section.
- A lightweight, rotating bobbin is present in the calibrated glass tube. It detects the amount of gas flowing through the flowmeter.
- Flowmeters of different gases are arranged in series and oxygen is the last gas to be added into the mixture (Fig. 42.1).

Common Outlet

Common outlet consists of 15 mm female connector to connect with the breathing system for safe delivery of anaesthetic gases to the patient. The pressure at this point is near atmospheric pressure (range 1–8 kPa).

ANAESTHETIC VAPOURIZERS

Vapourizer converts liquid inhalational anaesthetic agent into vapour under a controlled condition and adds to the fresh gas flow.

- Vaporizers can be draw over or plenum type. Draw over is low resistance vaporizer and, therefore, can be mounted within the breathing system.
- **Plenum vapourizer:**
  - It is high resistance and agent-specific vapourizer. It is mounted outside the breathing system.

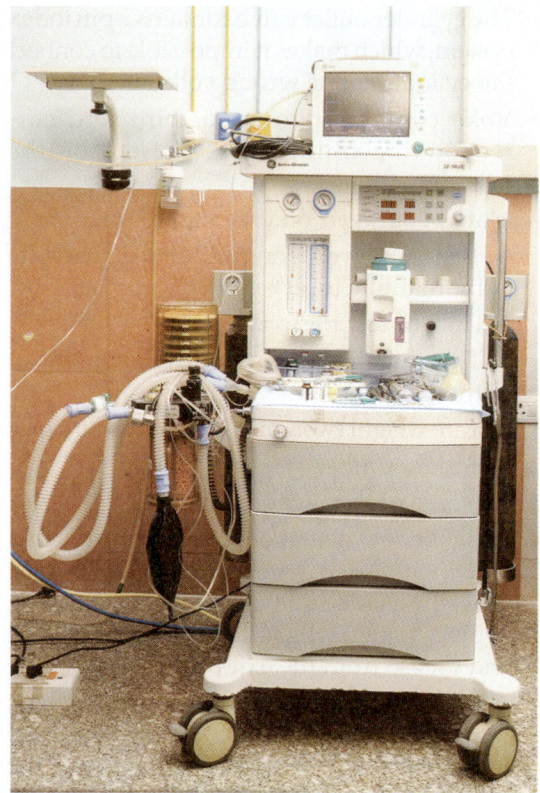

Fig. 42.1: Anaesthesia workstation

- As carrier gas passes through the vapourizer, it splits into two parts. One part enters into vapourization chamber and other part bypasses it.
- A portion of carrier gas entering into vapourization chamber is saturated with an inhalational anaesthetic agent. As it comes out from the vapourization chamber, it is mixed with rest of fresh gas and finally coming out from the common outlet.
- The vapourizer is thermocompensated and barocompensated. Thermocompensation is achieved by bimetallic strip.

ANAESTHETIC BREATHING SYSTEM

- Breathing systems deliver oxygen and anaesthetic gases and eliminate carbon dioxide.

- Breathing system consists of breathing hoses (corrugated 22 mm diameter non-kinkable tube), reservoir bag, adjustable pressure limiting (APL) valve (Fig. 42.2).

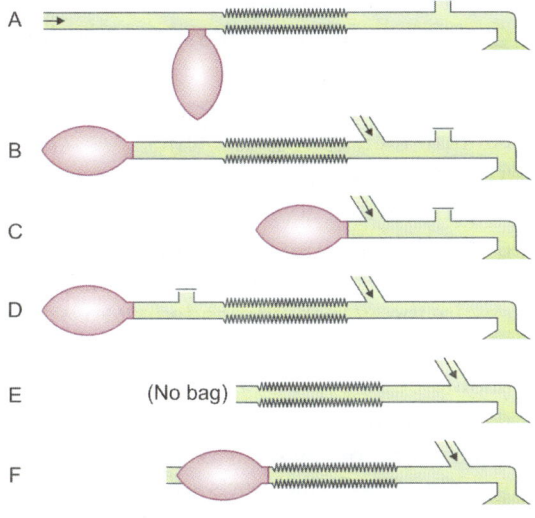

Fig. 42.2: Breathing system

- **Mapleson classification of breathing system:**
  - Breathing system is classified into A, B, C, D, E and F type of Mapleson system. Presently A, D, E, F and their modifications are used in clinical practice.
  - Mapleson A breathing system is also known as Magill system. It is very efficient for spontaneous ventilation but not suitable for controlled ventilation. It is not used in the paediatric population.
  - **Bain breathing system:** It is a coaxial breathing system, modifications of the Mapleson D system. Fresh gas flows through the inner tube and expired gas comes out from the outer tube. It is a very efficient breathing system for controlled ventilation. The requirement of fresh gas flow is 70-100 ml/kg/min.
  - **T piece system:** It is a modification of the Mapleson E and F system. Commonly used for paediatric patients. It is a valveless breathing system and offers minimal resistance to expiration.

- **Circle breathing system with soda lime:**
  - In the circle breathing system, expired gases are not voided in the atmosphere. The same gases are passed through soda lime to absorb carbon dioxide, then added to fresh gas and recycled for subsequent inspiration.
  - There is minimal loss of anaesthetic agents and causes minimum operation theatre pollution.
  - The circle system has seven components:
    - A fresh gas inflow source
    - Inspiratory and expiratory unidirectional valves
    - Inspiratory and expiratory corrugated tubes
    - Y piece connector
    - APL valve
    - Reservoir bag
    - Soda lime canister
  - Unidirectional valves are placed in the system to ensure unidirectional flow of gas.
  - Circle system can be used for spontaneous as well as controlled ventilation.

ANAESTHETIC VENTILATORS

Anaesthesia ventilators are used to provide intermittent positive pressure ventilation during general anaesthesia with muscular relaxation.

Classifications of Ventilators

- **Volume-cycled ventilator:** Tidal volume as set by anaesthesiologist is delivered during inspiration. Expiration starts after delivery of preset tidal volume.
- **Time-cycled ventilator:** Respiratory rate and inspiratory-expiratory ratio are set by anaesthesiologist. Thus the time of inspiration and expiration is fixed.
- **Pressure-cycled ventilator:** When the predetermined pressure is reached during inspiration, the ventilator switches over to expiration.

- **Flow-cycled ventilator:** When the pre-determined flow is reached, inspiration ends and expiration starts.

Source of power: Anaesthesia ventilators are usually electrically or pneumatically operated.

Manley Ventilator

- It is a time-cycled ventilator. It delivers all fresh gas flow in one minute divided in set tidal volume.
- Anaesthesia machine delivers fresh gas flow to the ventilator by a rubber tube.
- There are two bellows. Small bellow receives fresh gas flow and emptied into the main bellow. The main bellow finally delivers gases to the patient.
- It can be used for manual ventilation or controlled ventilation.

Bag in Bottle Ventilator

- It is a time-cycled ventilator.
- Bellow or bag is present within the chamber or bottle.
- Fresh gas is present within the bellows, whereas driving gas or compressed gas is within the chamber.
- Driving gas within the chamber compresses the bellow and delivers fresh gas to the patient.

PRE-ANAESTHETIC CHECKLIST

- A source of oxygen and device for manual ventilation is available in functional status. It is back up system in case of failure of the anaesthesia machine.
- Check and confirm that the suction machine is functioning.
- Check monitors and alarm systems and confirm their functional status.
- Turn on anaesthesia delivery system and confirm its functional status.
- Check the pressure of the oxygen cylinder attached to the anaesthesia machine and ensure the availability of adequate oxygen.
- Check the pressure in gas pipelines. It should be 50 psi.
- Confirm that vapourizers are properly attached at the back bar of the anaesthesia machine. Check filler parts are tightly closed.
- Confirm that no leak is present between the flowmeter and common gas outlet.
- Verify calibration of oxygen monitor and check the low oxygen alarm.
- Confirm that carbon dioxide absorbent is not exhausted.
- Perform leak test for breathing system.
- Confirm ventilator settings and functional status.

CHAPTER **43**

Monitoring and Recording of Vital Signs

Vital signs: The temperature, pulse, blood pressure, and respiration are called vital signs because:

- These signs are governed by vital organs.
- Changes in the condition of the patient, improvement or deterioration can be detected by monitoring these signs.

BODY TEMPERATURE

It is defined as the degree of heat maintained by the human body. The normal body temperature is 98.4°F or 37°C. Body temperature is measured by a clinical thermometer.

Indications

- Routine assessment of vital signs
- A patient suffering from fever (raised temperature)
- During the perioperative period

Procedure

- Explain the procedure and request for cooperation.
- Put the glass thermometer in disinfectant solution and then wash with plain water.
- Wipe thermometer with a clean cotton swab.

- Hold the thermometer between thumb and forefinger at the tip of the stem and shake it to drop the mercury level below 35°C.
- **Check temperature:**
  - *Oral method:* Place the bulb of a thermometer at the base of the tongue and ask the patient to close the lip for 2–3 minutes.
  - *Rectal method:*
    - Put on clean gloves and apply lubricant on the bulb of the thermometer.
    - Expose anus and ask the patient to breathe deeply. Insert a thermometer into the anus for 3 to 3.5 cm.
    - Keep it for two minutes.
  - *Axillary method:*
    - Place the bulb at the centre of the axilla and hold it tightly by keeping arm beside the chest.
    - Keep the thermometer in place for 3 minutes.
- Remove thermometer and wipe out with a sterile cotton ball.
- Hold the thermometer at eye level and note the temperature.
- Clean thermometer with soap and water and then dip in a disinfectant solution.

PULSE

There is expansion and recoil of an artery due to waves of blood as it forced through it, which makes pulsatile waves and felt as the pulse. The pulse can be felt by placing the finger on the artery where it is closed to the surface of the skin.

A pulse may be felt on the following points (Fig. 43.1).

- **Radial artery:** In front of the wrist at the base of the thumb.
- **Temporal artery:** Superior and lateral to the angle of the eye.
- **Carotid artery:** In between the trachea and sternocleidomastoid muscle.
- **Brachial artery:** Above the elbow in the antecubital fossa.

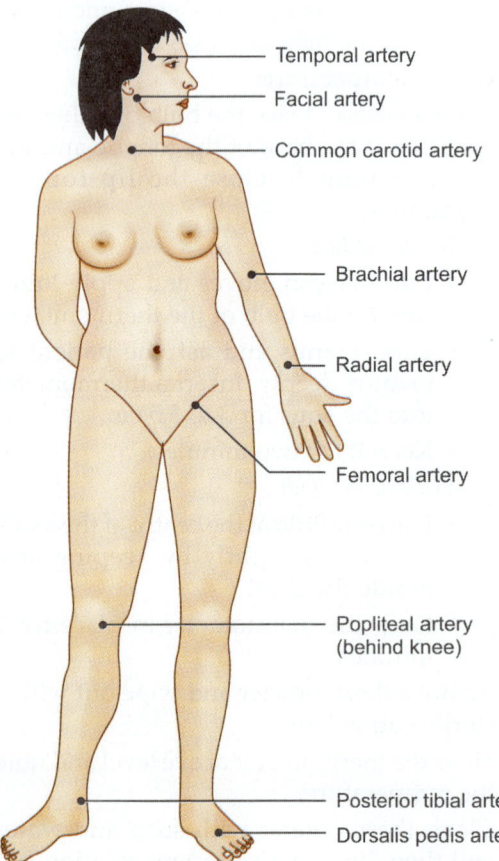

Fig 43.1: Location of finger to feel different pulse

- **Femoral artery:** Below inguinal ligament midway between the symphysis pubis and anterior superior iliac spine.
- **Popliteal artery:** Popliteal fossa at the back of the knee.
- **Dorsalis pedis artery:** At the dorsum of the foot, between extensor tendons of the great toe and second toe.
- **Posterior tibial artery:** On the medial surface of the ankle behind the medial malleolus.

Pulse Rate

Normal Rate

- **Adult:** 70 to 80 beat per minute
- **Old age:** 60 to 70 beat per minute
- **Newborn:** 130 to 140 beat per minute
- **Children:** 80 to 90 beat per minute

Assessment of Pulse

Pulse is checked to assess rate (beat per minute), rhythm (regular or irregular) and volume of the pulse. It helps to assess the circulatory status of the patient.

Procedure

- Explain the procedure to the patient.
- For assessment of radial pulse, keep arm of the patient on the side with palm facing downward.
- Palpate and check the pulse by placing three fingers on the pulse.
- Count the pulse for one minute.
- Assess rate, rhythm, volume, and condition of vessel walls.
- Record the pulse at regular intervals.

RESPIRATION

Respiration is the process of taking in oxygen and giving out carbon dioxide. It consists of inspiration, expiration, and pause.

- Respiration is assessed to determine the rate, rhythm, depth, and easiness of respiration.
- Respiratory rate varies according to the age of the patient. The normal respiratory rate

of a newborn baby is 30–40 breaths per minute. It gradually reduces to attain the normal respiratory rate of an adult, i.e. 14–16 breaths per minute.

- Depth of respiration determines the tidal volume of a person. Normal tidal volume is 7–8 ml/kg body weight.

Purpose of Assessment of Respiration

- To determine the rate of respiration
- To determine the regularity or rhythm of respiration.
- To assess the easiness of respiration
- To observe the movement of the muscles of the chest, nose, and abdomen.
- To monitor the position of the patient during breathing.

Procedure

- Allow the patient to attain either a sitting or supine position.
- Wait for 5 to 10 minutes to make him relaxed.
- Keep the hand of the patient over his lower part of the chest or abdomen.
- Keep fingers on the wrist of the patient as if checking the pulse and keep on eye to watch respiratory movements.
- Observe a few respiratory cycles to analyze depth and rhythm.
- See for any signs of respiratory obstruction such as noisy breathing, retraction of the chest wall or use of accessory muscles.
- Count respirations for one minute to assess the respiratory rate.
- Record findings related to respiration.

BLOOD PRESSURE

It is the force exerted by blood against the walls of the artery. The pressure exerted at the time of ventricular systole is called systolic blood pressure and exerted at the time of ventricular diastole is called diastolic blood pressure.

The average blood pressure of a healthy adult is 120/80 mm Hg. It is measured by a sphygmomanometer.

Purposes

- To determine blood pressure during the first visit at OPD or on admission for indoor patients and record as a baseline vital parameter.
- To determine the haemodynamic status of patients.
- To monitor the patient in the perioperative period as one of the vital parameters related to the cardiovascular system.
- To assess the effect of medical therapy in hypertensive patients.

Articles

- The sphygmomanometer consists of:
  - Blood pressure compression bag of appropriate size (width of compression bag should be 20% greater than the diameter of the extremity).
  - An inflation bulb (to raise the pressure of blood pressure cuff).
  - A manometer for measuring the pressure inside the cuff. There are two types of pressure manometer—mercury and aneroid manometer.
  - Screw type release valve for inflation and deflation of compression bag.
- Stethoscope

Procedure

- Explain the procedure and reassure the patient.
- Position the sphygmomanometer at the level of the heart of the patient.
- Select a cuff of appropriate size.
- Apply cuff about 2.5 cm above the point where the brachial artery is palpable.
- Fix the blood pressure cuff in such a way that the middle part of the rubber bladder should remain over the artery.
- The arm of the patient should be supported and at the level of the heart.

- Palpate the radial pulse and inflate the blood pressure cuff until the radial pulse disappears.
- Raise the cuff pressure 20–30 mm Hg beyond the point where pulse disappears.
- Gradually deflate the cuff and note the point at which pulse reappears.
- Place the diaphragm of the stethoscope on the brachial artery. Raise the pressure of the cuff up to the same point as done on previous occasions.
- Gradually deflate the cuff at a rate of 2–4 mm Hg per second.
- The appearance of the first sound should be noted as systolic blood pressure.
- The pressure measured by the sphygmomanometer should be noted as diastolic blood pressure when Korotkoff sound disappears or muffles.
- Deflate the cuff completely and remove from the arm of the patient.

INTAKE AND OUTPUT CHART

Measurement and recording of total fluid intake and output in 24 hours to analyze the fluid balance of the patient (Table 43.1).

Purposes

- To assess the fluid balance and detect dehydration or overhydration.
- To assess kidney function.

Procedure

- Explain the entire procedure and ask for the cooperation of the patient.
- Measure all oral fluids before ingestion and record the volume of fluid intake.
  Example: Glassful water—200 ml
  Cupful liquid—120 ml
- Measure all fluid in a graduated container before giving it to the patient.
- Record in the proper column of intake and output chart.
- Similarly, the volume of urine voided during micturition is measured in the measuring container and recorded in the appropriate column of the chart.
- After 24 hours, calculate the total intake and output and analyze the balance sheet of intake and output.
- Assess the loss from drainage tube, if any, and add to the output chart.

Table 43.1		Intake and output chart						
Name			**Ward/bed no**			**Hosp IP no**		
Date	**Time**	**Intake**		**Output**			**Stool**	**Misc**
		Oral	**IV fluids started infused**	**Urine**	**Emesis**	**Other**		

CHAPTER 44

Assessment and Management of Haemorrhage

Haemorrhage or blood loss is an inevitable consequence of any surgery due to injuries of blood vessels like arteries, veins and capillaries during operative procedures.

CLASSIFICATIONS OF HAEMORRHAGE

- **Based on the source of bleeding:**
  - *Arterial haemorrhage:* The blood is bright red and spurts with each heartbeat.
  - *Venous haemorrhage:* The blood is dark red in colour. There is a steady and continuous loss of blood.
  - *Capillary haemorrhage:* Blood is red and slowly oozes out.

- **Based on the time of haemorrhage:**
  - *Primary haemorrhage:* Occurs at the time of injury or surgery.
  - *Reactionary haemorrhage:* It occurs within 24 hours after injury or surgery. Hypertension in the postoperative period, coughing, straining, vomiting or retching are the common causes of reactionary haemorrhage.
  - *Secondary haemorrhage:* It occurs 5 to 7 days after surgery due to sloughing of the wall of blood vessels following infection.

- **Based on the duration of haemorrhage:**
  - Acute haemorrhage
  - Chronic haemorrhage

- **Based on the nature of haemorrhage:**
  - *External haemorrhage or revealed haemorrhage:* Bleeding is visible such as bleeding due to open cut injury. Amount of blood loss is easy to assess in external haemorrhage.
  - *Internal haemorrhage or concealed haemorrhage:* Bleeding occurs within the cavities and cannot be seen exteriorly. It may occur following rupture of ectopic pregnancy, injury of spleen, liver, lungs, heart or major vessels leading to haemothorax or haemoperitonium. Amount of blood loss is difficult to assess and primarily based on clinical findings of haemorrhagic shock and ultrasonography findings.

HAEMORRHAGIC SHOCK

Significant blood loss causes a reduction of total blood volume and produces features of hypovolaemic shock or haemorrhagic shock; characterized by pallor, tachycardia and hypotension.

Assessment of Blood Loss

Amount of blood loss differs in different types of surgeries. It may vary in the same type of surgery required for different pathology or done by the different surgeons. It also depends upon the duration of surgery. Accidental injury of major blood vessels may cause sudden unusual blood loss. Therefore, constant monitoring and assessment of blood loss are essential during surgery.

Method of Assessment

- Size of clot gives a rough idea about the amount of blood loss. A clenched fist size of clot is equal to 500 ml of blood loss.
- Blood loss following major fracture:
  - Tibia fracture causes about 500 to 1500 ml of blood loss.
  - Femur fracture causes 750 to 2000 ml of blood loss.
  - Pelvis fracture causes 1000 to 3000 ml of blood loss.
- Weight of dry swabs is subtracted from the weight of same swabs after mopping the surgical field flooded with blood. The difference in weight of swabs in gram is multiplied by 1½ to get the volume of blood loss during surgery.

The total amount of blood loss in ml
= Difference in weight of swab before and after use in gram × 1.5
- Measurement of volume of blood in the suction apparatus
- Measurement of CVP and estimations of haemoglobin and packed cell volume.
- Estimation of blood loss by assessing signs of haemorrhagic shock.

Depending upon the clinical signs and symptoms, the severity of haemorrhagic shock can be assessed and the amount of blood loss can be detected (Table 44.1).

MANAGEMENT OF HAEMORRHAGE

- **The arrest of haemorrhage:**
  - *External haemorrhage:* Remember three "Ps"—pressure, patience and packing
    - Apply pad and bandage to create pressure on the bleeding point.
    - Direct digital pressure on the artery supplying the area of injury and thus produces temporary arrest of haemorrhage.
    - Elevation of injured limb controls venous haemorrhage.
    - Application of tourniquet: Helps to control severe haemorrhage until some definite measures are taken.

Table 44.1	Classification of haemorrhagic shock			
	Class I	Class II	Class III	Class IV
Blood loss (ml)	<750	750–1500	1500–2000	>2000
Blood loss (%BV)	<15	15–30	30–40	>40
Pulse rate (bpm)	<100	>100	>120	>140
Systolic blood pressure (mm Hg)	N	N	↓	↓
Pulse pressure (mm Hg)	N	↓	↓↓	↓↓
Respiratory rate (breath/min)	14–20	20–30	30–40	>40
Urine output (ml/hour)	>30	20–30	5–15	Nil
Mental status	Anxious	Anxious	Confused	Lethargy

N= Normal, ↓ = fall, ↓↓ = severe fall

- Surgical ligation of bleeders
- Coagulation of bleeding points by electrocautery or diathermy.

– *Internal haemorrhage:* Surgical exploration, identification of bleeding points and check to bleed by direct pressure, ligation, cautery or some other way.

- Laparotomy for injury of liver, spleen, bowel or major vessels and control of bleeding by suturing, ligation of bleeders or splenectomy.
- Intercostal tube placement in cases of haemothorax.
- Internal pressure by inflation of balloon such as in case of bleeding oesophageal varices.
- Exploration, identification of bleeders and ligation.

- For local oozing, gauze soaked with adrenaline may be helpful.
- Bone wax to control oozing from bone

- **Restoration of lost blood volume:**
  – Intravenous cannulation with wide bore IV cannula and rapid infusion of crystalloids such as Ringer lactate and colloids to restore blood volume.
  – Blood transfusion, if blood loss is more than 20% or haemoglobin level is <7 gm%.
  – Prevention of coagulopathy especially after massive transfusion by the administration of platelet and fresh frozen plasma.

- **Supportive therapy:**
  – Raised foot end to increase venous drainage from lower limbs.
  – Oxygen therapy
  – Resuscitative measures, if the patient is in critical condition.

CHAPTER 45

Common Procedures: Intravenous Cannulation, Insertion of Nasogastric Tube and Urinary Catheterization

PERIPHERAL INTRAVENOUS CANNULATION

An intravenous cannula is inserted into a peripheral vein using aseptic technique. Intravenous cannulation is essential prior to any surgical procedure.

Purpose of Cannulation

- To provide fluid therapy during the perioperative period.
- To administer intravenous anaesthetic agents for induction and maintenance of anaesthesia.
- To administer emergency drugs to cope up any emergency during surgery.

Articles

- IV fluid
- IV administration set
- IV cannula
- IV stand
- IV start kit (includes antiseptic swab, tape, transparent dressing, tourniquet)
- Sterile gloves
- Towel/pad
- Arm splint

Procedure

- Open and prepare infusion set
  - Incise the packet and take out the IV infusion set.
  - Remove protective cover from the entry point of intravenous fluid bottle/bag.
  - Prime the tubing and remove air bubbles.
  - Hang the IV bottle with an infusion set on the IV stand.
- Prepare the patient by explaining the entire procedure. Explain that venipuncture may cause mild discomfort for a few seconds.
- Select the venipuncture site preferably on the nondominant arm of the patient. Choose the vein that is relatively straight and away from the wrist and elbow. Common sites for venipuncture are the inner arm, dorsal surface of the hand and dorsal surface of foot.
- Dilate the vein by:
  - Applying a tourniquet firmly about 15 cm above the venipuncture site
  - Massage/stroke the vein distal to the site
  - Encourage patient to clench and un-clench the fist
- Wash hands and put on gloves
- Clean venipuncture site by antiseptic swab

- **Insert intravenous cannula:**

  - Use non-dominant hand and stretch the skin below the venipuncture site.

  - Insert the IV cannula either by indirect method or direct method (Fig. 45.1).

  - *Indirect method:* Insert the IV cannula into the subcutaneous space directly parallel to the side of the vein. Gently move the tip of the needle toward the vein and gently pierce the vein. Fix the needle and gently advance the cannula into the vein.

  - *Direct method:* Hold the IV cannula with the bevel facing upward and at a 15–25° angle to the skin. Once cannula pierces the skin, it should be lower down to make it almost parallel and then pierce the vein. Loss of resistance may be felt. Advance the cannula within the venous lumen.

  - Withdraw the needle including protective cap over the needle adaptor and attach to the tubing of drip set. Start infusion slowly.

- Fix the catheter by adhesive tape.

- Dress the venipuncture site by a transparent dressing. Loop the drip set tubing on the extremity and secures it with tape.

- It may be connected with a syringe pump or infusion pump for slow and steady infusion at a constant rate.

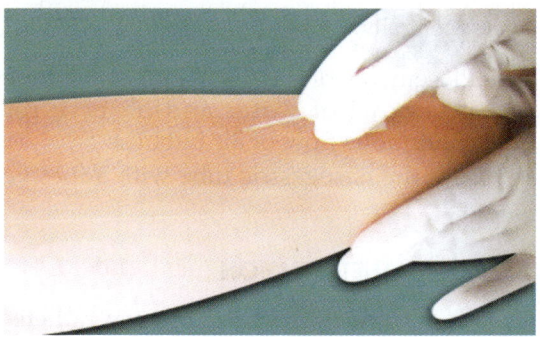

Fig. 45.1: Insertion of IV cannula

Complications

- Thrombophlebitis
- Extravasation of fluid

CENTRAL VENOUS CANNULATION

Cannulation of central veins, such as a right internal jugular vein or subclavian vein is indicated in the following situations:

- To measure central venous pressure
- To administer drugs in the central vein
- To provide parenteral nutrition

Articles

Same as peripheral venous cannulation except central venous cannula is used in place of routine IV cannula.

Procedure

- Prepare infusion set, obtain informed consent from the patient, wash hands and clean puncture site same as peripheral venous cannulation.

- Common vein for central venous cannulation is the right internal jugular vein because it is relatively straight on the right side. The subclavian vein is also used especially for long-term use.

- Position of the patient: Head down tilt and the head rotated to the left.

- Site of needle puncture: Midway between a line joining the mastoid process and sternoclavicular joint.

- Insert the needle at 45° angle and advance towards the right nipple to enter the vein.

- Insert the guidewire through the needle and remove the needle.

- Pass cannula over the guidewire.

- Position of the cannula should be checked by radiograph to ensure that its tip lies above the pericardial reflection.

- Use of ultrasonography has made the technique easy and has improved the success rate.

Complications

- Haemorrhage
- Air embolism
- Pneumothorax
- Thromboembolism
- Damage to other structures in the neck

INSERTION OF A NASOGASTRIC TUBE

The nasogastric tube is inserted into the stomach through nostril via nasopharynx and oesophagus. It is utilized to:

- Remove fluids and gas from the stomach (decompression of stomach)
- Feed the patient who cannot take orally but the gastrointestinal function is normal.
- Administer medicine
- Obtain specimen of gastric contents for laboratory studies
- Do gastric lavage

Articles

- Kidney tray
- Towel
- Sterile gauze piece
- Ryles tube
- Water-soluble lubricant
- Syringe (10 or 20 ml)
- Glass of water
- Adhesive tape and scissors
- Gloves

Procedure

- Explain the procedure to the patient and take consent.
- Turn the patient supine on the bed with a raised head end side.
- Wash hands and put on gloves
- To place the tip of the nasogastric tube at the stomach, approximate length can be estimated. Measure the length from the tip of the nose to the ear lobe and then to the tip of the xiphoid process. Mark the length with adhesive tape (Fig. 45.2).

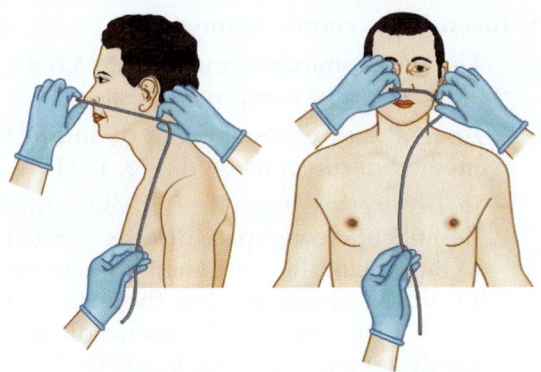

Fig. 45.2: Measuring length of the nasogastric tube

- Lubricate the tip of the tube with water-soluble lubricant using a sterile gauze piece.
- Insert the tube through the nostril towards backward and downward to reach nasopharynx.
- Flex the head of the patient towards the chest after the tube is passed nasopharynx.
- Ask the patient to take sips of water and swallow on command. Advance nasogastric tube 3–4 inches when the patient swallows. Continue the process until it reaches up to the designated mark.
- Do not push the tube, if there is resistance or signs of distress such as coughing, straining or cyanosis. Pull back the tube for some length, relieve the distress and reinsert after some time.
- Check the placement of the tip of the tube in the stomach by:
  - Aspiration of gastric content with a syringe, or
  - Placements of the distal end of the tube in a bowl of water and observe for continuous flow of air bubbles.
- Secure the nasogastric tube with adhesive tape.

URINARY CATHETERIZATION

It is the introduction of the urinary catheter through the urethra into the urinary bladder to drain urine from the bladder.

Purposes

For Intermittent Catheterization

- To relieve bladder distension
- To empty bladder prior to surgery of rectum, vagina or other pelvic organs. This prevents accidental injury of the distended bladder.
- To measure the amount of residual urine when the bladder is incompletely emptied.

For Indwelling Catheterization

- To facilitate continuous drainage of urine from the bladder after injury or surgery on the urinary tract.
- To prevent urine contamination of a wound such as repair of the perineum.
- To manage incontinence of urine, when other measures fail (failure of condom drainage).

Articles

- The sterile tray containing sterile gloves, towel, the catheter (indwelling/straight catheter of appropriate size), cotton swabs and bowl with an antiseptic solution.
- A sterile syringe filled with distilled water
- Spotlight
- Adhesive tape and scissors
- Water-soluble lubricant

Procedure

- Explain the procedure, take consent and request for cooperation.
- Maintain privacy with a temporary partition or curtain. Expose only the needed parts.
- Assemble the articles at the bedside before starting the procedure.
- **Position of the patient:**
  - *Female:* Supine position with knees flexed and thigh externally rotated
  - *Male:* Supine position with the abduction of the thigh.

- The clean perineal area with soap and water
- Adjust spotlight
- Wash hands and put on gloves
- Pour the antiseptic solution into a bowl. Use a correct concentration of antiseptic solution which is safe for skin and mucous membrane. The area around the urethral meatus is cleaner than anus. Therefore, cleaning should be started from urethral area and gradually approach towards anal region to prevent unnecessary contaminations.
- Open the outer cover of the catheter pack and place the catheter on the sterile tray.
- Lubricate the tip of the catheter liberally with a water-soluble lubricant.
- **Catheterization of a female patient** (Fig. 45.3):
  - Retract labia fully with nondominant hand and expose urethral meatus.
  - Hold the catheter near the tip with the dominant hand and introduce gently through meatal opening.
  - Length of the urethra is approximately 3 to 5 cm. Once the tip enters into the bladder, urine begins to flow and appears at the distal opening of the catheter.

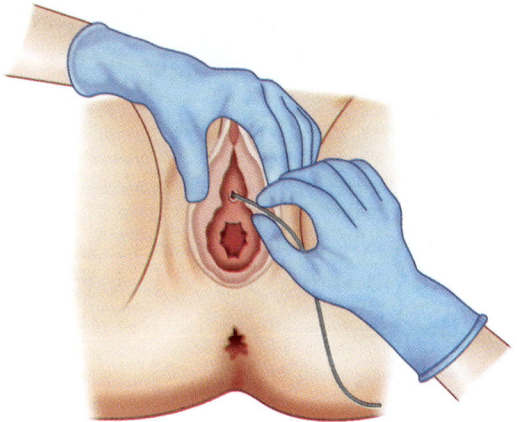

Fig. 45.3: Insertion of a urinary catheter in a female patient

- **Catheterization of a male patient** (Fig. 45.4):
  - Grasp the penis firmly below glans and retract the foreskin with the nondominant hand.
  - Hold the catheter near the tip with the dominant hand and gently introduce through the meatal opening.

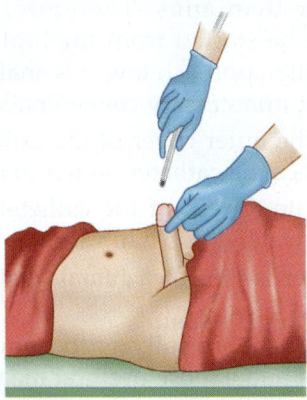

Fig. 45.4: Insertion of a urinary catheter in a male patient

- Insert catheter for 15 to 25 cm until urine begins to flow.
- The patient must be relaxed during the procedure. They may be asked to take deep breaths.
- The gentle insertion of the catheter is necessary to prevent injury to the mucous membrane. Do not force to introduce the catheter.
- Collect all urine in a sterile kidney tray and remove the catheter in case of intermittent catheterization.
- **For indwelling catheterization:**
  - Introduce sterile distilled water to inflate the balloon.
  - Pull catheter gently outward and connect the other end of the catheter to urosac (urine collecting bag) for collection of urine.
  - Fix the catheter to the thigh of the patient with adhesive tape.

CHAPTER 46

Oxygen Therapy

Oxygen is an essential element for the survival of every living organism. Human beings breathe in air, which contains 21% oxygen and breathes out carbon dioxide. If this process is inadequate to fulfill the requirement of oxygen, its level in the blood decreases and the patient needs supplemental oxygen.

PURPOSE OF OXYGEN THERAPY

Oxygen therapy is the administration of oxygen at concentrations greater than that in the air to treat or prevent hypoxaemia (not enough oxygen in the blood).

The purpose of oxygen therapy is to increase oxygen saturation in tissues, where the oxygen level is low due to illness or injury.

Important Basic Parameters Related to Oxygen (Normal Values)

- FiO_2 (fractional oxygen concentration in inspired air)—21%
- PaO_2 (partial pressure of oxygen in arterial blood)—98–100 mm Hg
- PvO_2 (partial pressure of oxygen in venous blood)—40 mm Hg
- SaO_2 (arterial oxygen saturation or amount of oxygenated haemoglobin in the blood)—100%

OBJECTIVES OF OXYGEN THERAPY

- To correct documented or suspected hypoxaemia
  - PaO_2 < 60 mm Hg or SaO_2 <90% at room air

    or

  - PaO_2 or SaO_2 below desirable range for a specific clinical scenario.
- To reduce the symptoms associated with chronic hypoxaemia.
- To decrease the workload that hypoxaemia imposes on the cardiopulmonary system.

Assessment of Hypoxia

- **ABG monitoring:** To assess PaO_2
- **Pulse oximetry:** To assess SaO_2
- **Clinical assessment to find out features of hypoxia:**
  - *Central nervous system:* Confusion, restlessness, disorientation
  - *Cardiovascular system:* Tachycardia, hypertension followed by bradycardia, hypotension, and arrhythmia
  - *Respiratory system:* Dyspnoea, laboured breathing
  - *Skin:* Cyanosis

OXYGEN THERAPY DEVICES

Variable Performance Devices

Inspired oxygen concentration (FiO_2) is variable and depends upon the inspiratory flow rate, oxygen flow rate and the duration of the expiratory pause.

- No reservoir capacity: Nasal cannula/nasal prongs
- Small reservoir capacity: Mask
- Large reservoir capacity: Mask with a bag

Fixed Performance Devices

They provide accurate inspired oxygen concentration and do not depend upon the ventilation of the patient because fresh gas flow is higher than the inspiratory flow rate.

- HAFOE system (high airflow oxygen enrichment device): Ventimask
- Ventilators
- Anaesthesia machine with the breathing system

Oxygen Therapy by Nasal Cannula/Nasal Prongs

Articles Required

- **Oxygen source:** Oxygen cylinder or oxygen gas pipeline
- A nasal cannula or nasal prongs with connecting tubes (Fig. 46.1)
- Humidifier with distilled water (Fig. 46.2)
- Flowmeter (Fig. 46.2)
- Gauze pads, adhesive tape, etc.

Procedure

- Explain the procedure to patients and relatives and answer all relevant questions asked by them.
- Thoroughly wash both hands.
- Set up oxygen equipment including humidifier in the following steps.
  - Attach flowmeter to the source of oxygen (gas pipelines or cylinder) and set the flow meter at 'off' position.
  - Fill up the humidifier with sterile water up to the level marked on it.
  - Attach humidifier to the flowmeter.
  - Attach nasal cannula with a connecting tube to the humidifier.
  - Set the flowmeter to supply oxygen at a rate prescribed by the doctor.
  - Ensure uninterrupted flow of oxygen by checking bubbles in the humidifier or feeling the flow of oxygen at the outlet.
- Insert tips of the cannula to nares of the patient and adjust straps around-ear for proper fitting.
- Encourage the patient to breathe through the nose with a closed mouth.

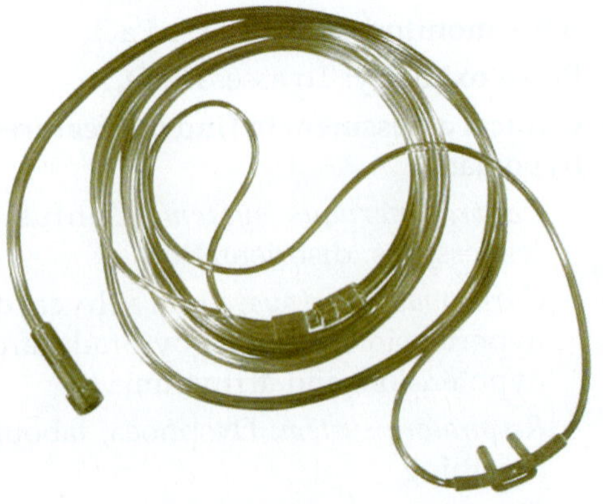

Fig. 46.1: Nasal prongs

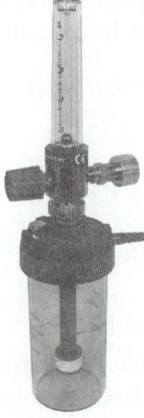

Fig. 46.2: Oxygen flowmeter including humidifier

- Monitor the equipment at regular intervals and ensure uninterrupted oxygen supply.
- Oxygen concentration at inspired air at different oxygen flow rates by nasal cannula.

Oxygen flow rate (L/min)	FiO_2 (fraction of oxygen at inspired gases)
1	0.24
2	0.28
3	0.32
4	0.36
5	0.40
6	0.44

OXYGEN THERAPY BY SIMPLE FACE MASK OR VENTURI MASK

- The nasal cannula is replaced by a face mask. Other parts of the oxygen therapy system remain the same.
- Mask is placed over the face of the patient. Space between the mask and face, in front of the nose and mouth, acts as a reservoir for oxygen and thus higher FiO_2 can be delivered.
- **Simple face mask:** FiO_2 0.35–0.55 can be delivered with an oxygen flow rate of 7–8 litre/minute (Fig. 46.3).

- **Venturi mask:** It works on the venturi principle. It consists of venturi valves of different diameters which are capable of delivering different concentrations of oxygen. Venturi valves are colour coded and can deliver FiO_2 from 0.24 to 0.60.
- **Partial rebreathing mask:** Face mask is connected with the reservoir bag. The flow of oxygen must be sufficient to prevent reservoir bag from deflating after inspiration. The oxygen flow rate of 6–10 litres per minute increases FiO_2 to 0.50–0.70.
- **Nonrebreathing mask:** Face mask is connected with a reservoir bag containing a nonrebreathing valve. FiO_2 can be increased up to 0.70 to 1.0 with a fresh gas flow of 6–10 litres by this device (Fig. 46.3).

Articles Required

- **Oxygen sources:** Oxygen cylinder or oxygen gas pipeline
- Simple mask or venturi mask with or without reservoir bag
- Humidifier with distilled water
- Flowmeter
- Gauze pieces, adhesive tape, etc.

Procedure

- The procedure remains the same as done for oxygen therapy by nasal cannula except for a few differences.

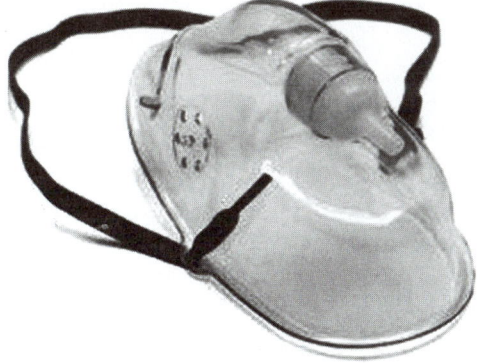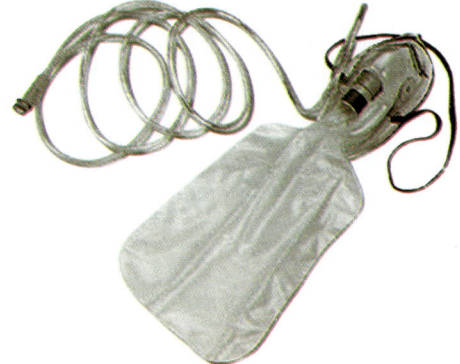

Fig. 46.3: Simple mask, venturi mask, and non-rebreathing mask

- In place of nasal cannula, face mask and connecting tubes are attached to the humidifier.
- Mask is placed on the face of the patient. It is applied from the nose downward. Fit the metal piece of the mask to conform to the shape of the nose.
- Apply an elastic band of face mask around the head of the patient and make it tight to reduce oxygen leakage.
- Monitor for uninterrupted oxygen flow from an oxygen device.

COMPLICATIONS OF OXYGEN THERAPY

- Oxygen toxicity
- Depression of ventilation
- Retinopathy of prematurity
- Absorption atelectasis
- Fire hazard

Precautions

- The goal of oxygen therapy is to use the lowest possible FiO_2 compatible with adequate tissue oxygenation.
- To prevent oxygen toxicity, it is recommended that;
  - 100% of FiO_2 should not be used for more than 12 hours.
  - 80% of FiO_2 should not be used for more than 24 hours.
  - 60% of FiO_2 should not be used for more than 36 hours.
- In patients with chronic lung disease such as COPD, oxygen should be used judiciously. The concentration of oxygen should be increased gradually and it should never be delivered more than 2–3 litres per minute.
- Finally, it must be remembered that oxygen is a drug. It is extremely beneficial when used appropriately. It is potentially harmful when misused or abused.

CHAPTER 47

Management of Airway

Airway management means the establishment and maintenance of patent airway in patients during general anaesthesia.

General anaesthesia produces various effects on the respiratory system, that include:

- Loss of airway patency
- Loss of protective airway reflexes
- Hypoventilation or apnoea

Therefore, the management of airway is one of the essential and most important steps of general anaesthesia.

TECHNIQUES OF MAINTAINING PATENT AIRWAY

- **"Sniffing the early morning air position":** To maintain a patent airway in an anaesthetized patient, displace the mandible anteriorly by holding the lower jaw and extend the neck at the atlanto-occipital joint.
- **Insertion of nasopharyngeal or oropharyngeal airway:** General anaesthesia produces relaxation of muscles of pharynx and floor of the mouth. Therefore, flaccid tongue falls back on the posterior pharyngeal wall and relaxation of muscles causes collapse of the upper airway.

Insertion of oropharyngeal and nasopharyngeal airway helps to keep the airway clear by displacing tongue.

OROPHARYNGEAL AIRWAY

- The oropharyngeal airway is available in different sizes for the different age group of patients from neonate to adult.
- The correct size of the airway should be chosen so that the tip of the airway must reach up to the posterior pharyngeal wall.
- Size of the airway can be assessed by placing the airway besides the face. Size of the airway such that it should extend from the angle of the mouth to the tragus (Fig. 47.1).

Technique

- Open the mouth by the left hand and assess for the presence of any secretions in the airway. Clear the secretion by suction using a sterile suction catheter.
- Hold the oropharyngeal airway by the right hand and slowly insert it inside the oral cavity with its concavity towards the palate.
- After insertion of 50% of airway inside the mouth, turn the airway 180° and move further to reach the tip up to the posterior pharyngeal wall.
- Observe for any signs of airway obstruction.
- Limitation: Oropharyngeal airway is poorly tolerated by conscious patients. The nasopharyngeal airway is better tolerated by conscious or semiconscious patients.

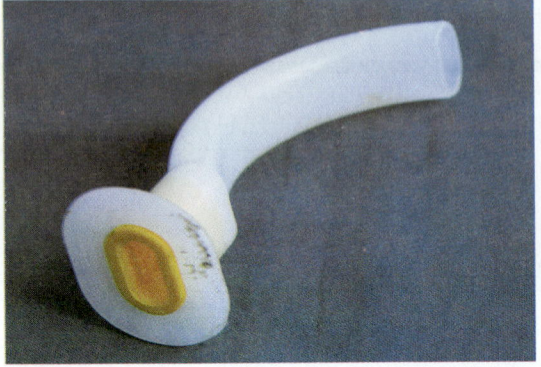

Fig. 47.1: Oropharyngeal airway

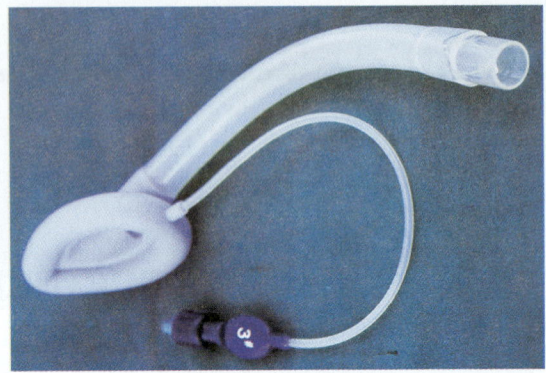

Fig. 47.2: Laryngeal mask airway

NASOPHARYNGEAL AIRWAY

- It is a soft tube made of latex or silicon. It is available in various sizes.
- Correct length of the airway can be chosen by placing it by the side of the face. It should extend from the nostril up to tragus.
- The diameter of the nasopharyngeal tube should be the same as the endotracheal tube for that patient.
- Lubricate the nasopharyngeal airway and insert gently through one of the nostrils until it reaches up to the posterior pharyngeal wall.
- Observe for any signs of airway obstruction.

SUPRAGLOTTIC DEVICES

- Supraglottic devices are very commonly used by anaesthesiologists during general anaesthesia for:
  - Maintenance of clear airway
  - Administration of inhalational anaesthetic agents
- Common supraglottic devices used by anaesthesiologists are Classic LMA, LMA Proseal, LMA fast trach, combitube, Cobra perilaryngeal airway, I-Gel, Baska mask, etc. (Fig. 47.2)

ENDOTRACHEAL INTUBATION

Passing of an endotracheal tube (slender hollow tube) into the trachea through nostril or mouth using aseptic technique to secure airway and facilitate artificial ventilation.

Indications

- To administer general anaesthesia for a long period (more than 1 hour)
- To protect the respiratory tract from aspiration
- To provide intermittent positive pressure ventilation
- To clear excessive secretions from the lungs.

Equipment

Laryngoscope

- It has two parts—handles and detachable blade.
- The handle is used to hold the laryngoscope. It contains batteries, which is a source of electricity for the bulb.
- The blade is attached to handle at a right angle to each other.
  - The blade has a flange to push the tongue towards the left side. This creates more room for visualization of glottis.

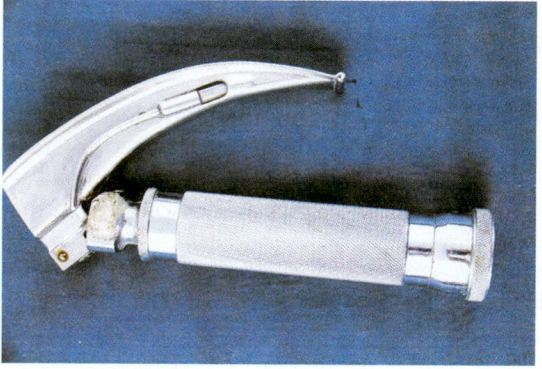

Fig. 47.3: Laryngoscope

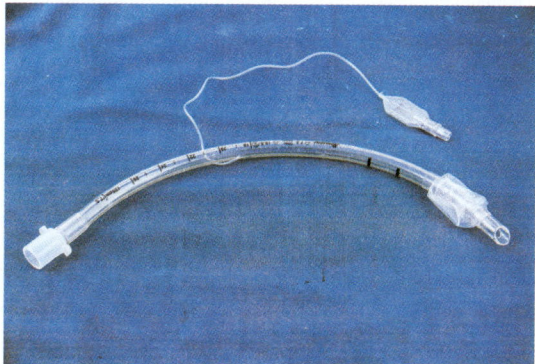

Fig. 47.4: Endotracheal tube

- At the tip of the blade, there is a bulb. It provides light for visualization of glottic-opening (Fig. 47.3).
- There are various types of laryngoscope:
  - **Macintosh laryngoscope:** Blade is curved. The commonest type of laryngoscope, used in adult patients.
  - **Miller laryngoscope:** Blade is straight. It is used in children.
  - **McCoy laryngoscope:** Blade has tilted movable tip, creates extra pressure at the base of the epiglottis to visualize glottis opening in difficult cases.
  - Bullard laryngoscope is used in patients with cervical spine immobility.
  - Short handled laryngoscope is used in obese patients and obstetric patients.

Endotracheal Tube (Fig. 47.4)

- It is a curved tube, commonly made up of polyvinyl chloride (PVC).
- It has two ends. Machine end is connected to a universal 15 mm diameter connector. The patient end is bevelled.
- An inflatable cuff is present near the patient end. It prevents aspiration and leakage of gases during artificial ventilation. The inflatable cuff is attached to a pilot balloon with a one-way valve. It is used to inflate the cuff.

- **Size of endotracheal tube:** Endotracheal tube is available in different sizes for the different age group of patients. Size of the endotracheal tube varies from 1.5 to 8.5 mm internal diameter.
- **Selection of endotracheal tube:**
  - *Adult male:* 8–8.5 mm
  - *Adult female:* 7–7.5 mm
  - *Preterm baby:* 2.5 mm or less
  - *Neonate:* 3 mm
  - *Children less than 6 years:* Age/3 + 3.5
  - *Children more than 6 years:* Age/4 + 4.5 (Fig. 47.4)

Role of an Assistant during Endotracheal Intubation

- Explain the procedure and take consent well in advance from a fully conscious patient.
- Place the patient in the supine position and keep a pillow (4–6 inch height) below the head.
- Remove denture and fix the loose teeth, if any.
- Once the patient is ventilated with oxygen using bag and mask, provide laryngoscope to anaesthesiologist for laryngoscopy.
- Keep ready sterile catheter attached to a suction machine for clearing secretions from the upper airway, if present.

- After visualization of glottis opening by an anaesthesiologist, provide the lubricated endotracheal tube with stilette *in situ*.
- Manipulate larynx by pressing thyroid cartilage backward, upward and right side (BURP) to improve visualization of glottis.
- After the introduction of the endotracheal tube, remove the stilette.
- Anaesthesiologist connects the endotracheal tube with a breathing bag or ventilator and starts ventilation.
- Verify the placement of a tube in the trachea by:
  - Bilateral movement of the chest with each inspiration.
  - Bilateral equal air entry on both sides of the lungs.
  - Confirmation by capnograph
- Secure the position of the endotracheal tube by adhesive tape.
- Inflate the cuff of the endotracheal tube with air.

DIFFICULT AIRWAY

Airway management with endotracheal intubation is a routine procedure for patients need general anaesthesia. It is safe and easy for the conventionally trained anaesthesiologist.

A difficult airway is defined as the clinical situation in which a conventionally trained anaesthesiologist experiences difficulty with face mask ventilation, difficulty in tracheal intubation or both.

The difficult airway can be predicted with a proper preoperative assessment of airway in the majority of cases. In a rare situation, preoperative airway assessment does not reveal any abnormality but the difficulty may be experienced during ventilation or intubation. This is called unanticipated difficult airway, a very serious clinical scenario.

To deal with a case of a difficult airway, "difficult airway trolley" must be kept ready in each operation theatre.

Difficult Airway Trolley

- It is a mobile trolley with a top workspace and 4 to 5 drawers.
- Difficult airway guidelines and locations of different types of equipment used in such scenario kept in different drawers must be written in bold letter and displayed on the trolley.

Equipment in Difficult Airway Trolley

- More than one laryngoscope:
  - Multiple sizes of Macintosh curved blade
  - Miller straight blade
  - McCoy blade
- Different sizes of the endotracheal tube
- Different sizes of Bougies and stiletto
- Aintree intubating catheter
- Different sizes of oropharyngeal and nasopharyngeal airway
- Different sizes of mask
- Supraglottic devices:
  - Intubating LMA
  - LMA proseal
  - LMA supreme
- Fibreoptic bronchoscopy with all accessories
- Equipment for the establishment of surgical airway:
  - Cricothyrotomy set
  - Needle cricothyrotomy + TTJV
  - Large cannulae cricothyrotomy
  - Surgical cricothyrotomy
- Instruments for anaesthesia of the upper airway:
  - Nebulizer
  - Atomizers
  - Xylocaine spray
  - Xylocaine 4% topical
  - Nasal decongestant
- Suction machine with a catheter

Difficult airway trolley should be checked regularly to analyze the functional status of different instruments.

CHAPTER 48

Incentive Spirometry, Chest Physiotherapy, Postural Drainage, and Nebulization Therapy

INCENTIVE SPIROMETER

Incentive spirometer encourages the patient to do respiratory exercise. It assists the patient in voluntary deep breathing.

Ball of incentive spirometer moves upward when patient takes deep breath. Movement of ball is visible to the patient and inspires to achieve better results. The incentive is to achieve a certain volume of air and hold it for 3 seconds (Fig. 48.1).

Purposes
- To improve pulmonary ventilation
- To expand collapsed alveoli
- To prevent postoperative respiratory complications
- To loosen secretions of the respiratory tract

Indications
- Postoperative patients
- Patients with obstructive and restrictive lung diseases
- Patients with prolonged immobilization and suffering from chronic debilitating diseases

Articles
- There are two types of incentive spirometer—volume spirometer and flow spirometer.

- **Volume spirometer:** Tidal volume of a spirometer is set and patient is asked to achieve the set target by deep breath. Set tidal volume is increased gradually step by step.
- **Flow spirometer:** The spirometer contains a number of movable balls. These balls are pushed up and kept them suspended by the force of the breath. The amount of air inhaled by the patient determines the number of balls remained suspended.

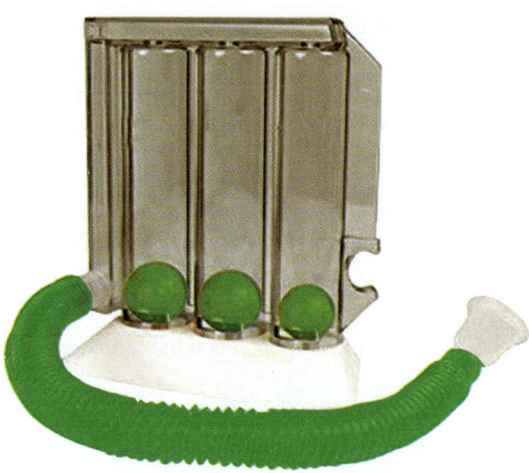

Fig. 48.1: Incentive spirometer

Procedure

- Explain the procedure and objectives of an incentive spirometer.
- Ask the patient to assume a semi-Fowler's or high-Fowler's position.
- Hold the spirometer in an upright position by one hand and hold mouthpiece with the other hand.
- Do not breathe through nose. Use nose clip, if necessary.
- Ask the patient to exhale normally and then keep lips tightly around the mouthpiece.
- Take breathing to elevate the balls and then hold the breath for 2 seconds.
- Gradually increase the duration up to 6 seconds.
- Remove lips from the mouthpiece than exhale normally.
- Continue same procedure several times as breathing exercise.

POSTURAL DRAINAGE

It is the gravitational clearance of secretions from different bronchial segments by acquiring a specific position.

For drainage from a specific tracheo-bronchial tree, a specific posture is adapted and chest physiotherapy is initiated (Table 48.1). Once secretion reaches into the trachea, it can be coughed out by the patient (Fig. 48.2).

Contraindications

- Increased intracranial pressure
- Head injury/spinal injury/rib fracture
- Bronchopleural fistula
- Empyema
- Active haemorrhage in the respiratory tract

Table 48.1	Position of the patient for postural drainage	
S. no.	Involved lobe of lung	Posture of patient
1.	Left and right upper lobe anterior apical bronchi	Sitting posture with leaning backward
2.	Left and right upper lobe posterior apical bronchi	Sitting posture with leaning forward on a pillow or cardiac table
3.	Left and right anterior upper lobe bronchi	Straight supine with a small pillow under knees
4.	Left upper lobe lingular bronchus	The patient lies down in right lateral position with raised foot end of bed 30 cm. Place pillow behind back and roll patient one-fourth on the pillow.
5.	Right middle lobe bronchus	The patient lies down in left lateral position with raised foot end of bed to 30 cm. Place pillow behind the back and roll patient one-fourth turned onto pillow.
6.	Left and right anterior lower lobe bronchi	The patient lies down supine with a pillow under the knees. The bed should be in a Trendelenburg position.
7.	Right lower lobe lateral bronchus	The patient lies down on left lateral position with foot end raised 45 to 50 cm
8.	Left lower lobe lateral bronchus	The patient lies down on right lateral position with foot end raised 45 to 50 cm
9.	Right and left lower lobe superior bronchi	The patient lies down on a prone position with pillow under the stomach
10.	Right and left posterior basal branch	The patient lies down on a prone position with foot end to be raised 45 cm (Trendelenburg position)

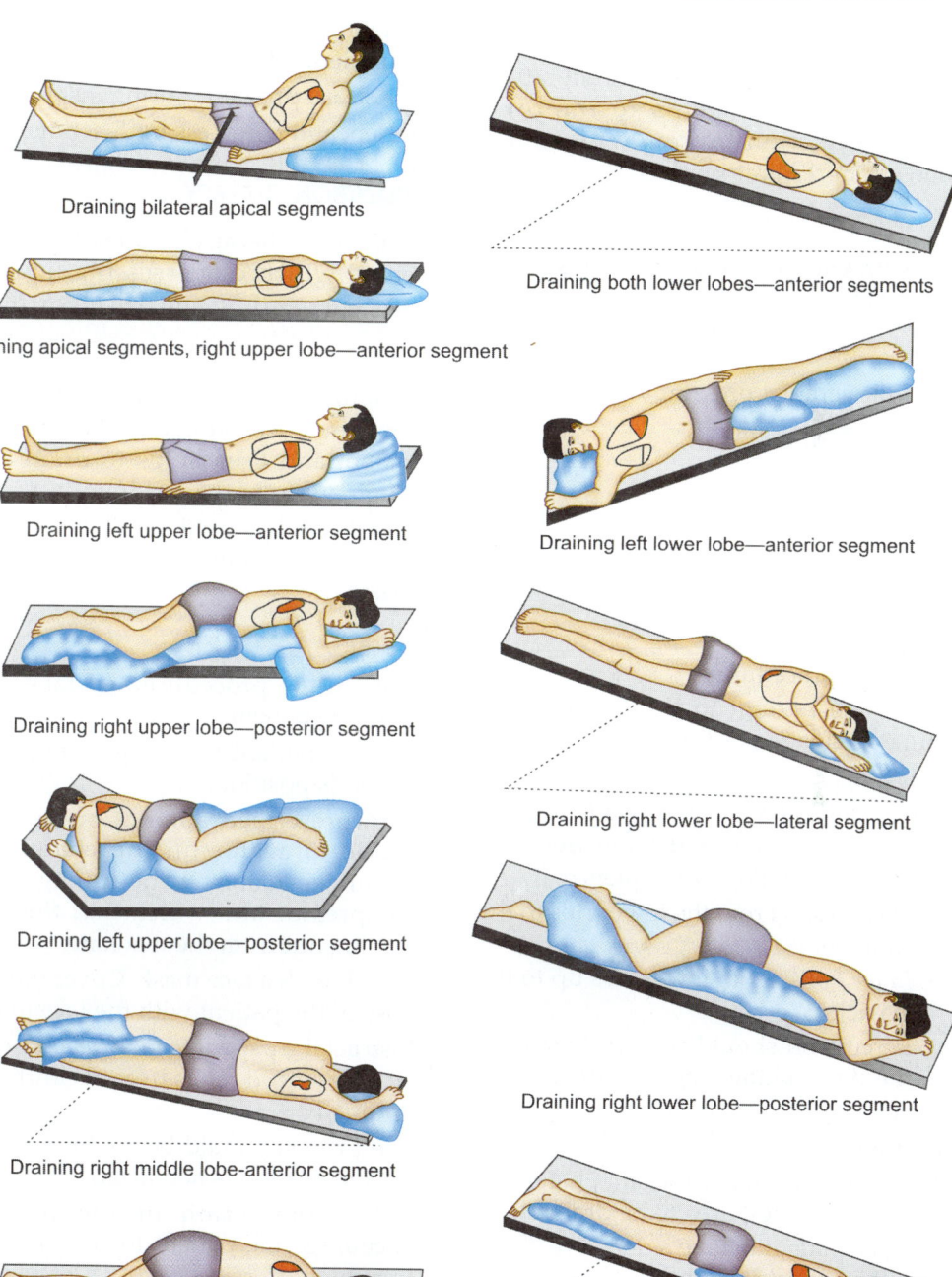

Draining bilateral apical segments

Draining apical segments, right upper lobe—anterior segment

Draining both lower lobes—anterior segments

Draining left upper lobe—anterior segment

Draining left lower lobe—anterior segment

Draining right upper lobe—posterior segment

Draining right lower lobe—lateral segment

Draining left upper lobe—posterior segment

Draining right middle lobe-anterior segment

Draining right lower lobe—posterior segment

Draining right middle lobe—posterior segment

Draining lower lobe—posterior segment

Fig. 48.2: Postural drainage

CHEST PHYSIOTHERAPY

It is the process of percussion and vibration over chest wall that helps to improve respiratory function by removing thick secretions from respiratory tract.

Indications

Patients with thick tenacious secretions in the respiratory tract.

Contraindications

- Raised intracranial pressure
- Painful chest condition
- Lung tumour
- Pneumothorax
- Haemoptysis
- Spinal injuries

Procedure

- Explain the procedures.
- Instruct the patient to lie down in the postural drainage position.
- **Percussion:**
  - Keep a towel on the chest wall.
  - Clap with the cupped hand over the chest wall in following sequence:
    - *On the back:* From the lower ribs to the shoulder
    - *In the front:* From lower ribs up to the clavicle
    - Percussion should not be done over the liver, kidney, spleen, breast and spine.
- **Vibration:**
  - Place one hand above the other hand and keep on the chest area to be drained.
  - Ask the patient to take a deep breathing and then exhale slowly.
  - Vibrate the palmar surface of hand with moderate force during expiration.
  - Release pressure during inspiration.
  - Repeat the process for 5–6 times.

NEBULIZATION THERAPY

Nebulization therapy is done by nebulizer machine which disperses the liquid into microscopic particles and delivers to the lung.

Uses

- Nebulization is used to liquefy the thick and tenacious secretions of the respiratory system and thus helps to drain and/or cough out from the respiratory system.
- Nebulization is used to deliver bronchodilators to the lungs and relieve bronchospasm.

Procedure

- Explain the procedure and take consent from the patient.
- Ask the patient to take a sitting or semi-Fowler's position.
- Add prescribed amount of medication, saline or water on the chamber of a nebulizer. Connect the tubing with the compressor and watch that fine mist is coming out from the machine.
- Attach with a face mask. Cover mouth and nose of the patient with the face mask.
- Instruct the patient to take deep inspiration slowly, hold the breath and expire gradually.
- The process should be continued until all the medication is nebulized.
- After completion of the procedure, encourage the patient to cough and deep breathing exercises.

CHAPTER 49

Surgical Dressing and Application of Plaster Slab

A surgical dressing is a procedure where the wound is covered with a sterile material aseptically. The basic idea of surgical dressing is to create an environment where both surgical and non-surgical wounds can heal without any complications like haemorrhage, flare-up or spread of infection and deep tissue necrosis.

Aseptic technique is important while applying or changing a dressing to avoid introducing infection into the wound.

If the wound is already infected, care should be taken to avoid further contamination with other organisms.

A surgical dressing is done usually in one corner of the ward where working space is available.

DRESSING TROLLEY

The materials and instruments required for dressing are kept in a dressing trolley specially designed for this purpose. The items in dressing trolley are:

- Dressing drum containing sterile gauze piece, cotton roll, bandage, and small draping material.
- Dressing sterile tray containing sponge holding forceps, artery forceps, thumb forceps, scissors, stitch cutting scissors,

needle holder, needle and suture materials, gauze piece, two small pots.
- The tray should be wrapped with a sterile linen piece. One complete dressing tray is used for dressing one wound. The number of dressing tray in the trolley depends on the volume of the patients.
- One wide-mouthed sterile bottle containing antiseptic lotion with a Cheattle forceps to hold and lift sterile material from one place to another.
- Povidone-iodine solution
- Rectified spirit
- Chlorhexidine solution
- Hydrogen peroxide
- Plaster of Paris bandage
- Disposable plastic bags
- Modern complete dressing materials with self-adhesive tape like semipermeable film dressing, hydrogel dressing, hydrocolloid dressing (for different wound conditions).
- Sterile gloves

DRESSING PROCEDURE

Step-1

- Dressing procedure has to be explained properly after identifying the patient and the wound.

- It is mandatory to see the direction of the physician regarding type of dressing or stitch removal.
- The privacy of the patient is maintained by using curtain or mobile screen.

Step-2

- Top of the dressing trolley with legs is cleaned with soap, water, and disinfectant. Hands are washed after wearing an apron.
- Nonsterile gloves are used for removing old dressing. The inner side of the dressing pad is inspected to see the colour and smell of the exudate, if any. Greenish smelling exudate indicates a Gram-negative infection of the wound. Yellowish pus is seen in pyogenic infection. A fresh blood comes from granulation tissue of the wound after removal of dressing.
- Sometimes removal of dressing is painful. If dressing is soaked with sterile normal saline, removal becomes easy and painless. Old dressings are disposed into a dirty clinical waste bag.

Step-3

- Hands are washed again and new sterile gloves are used for actual dressing.
- The assistant will open the dressing tray and the trolley top is covered with a sterile piece of cloth kept in the tray.
- The tray is kept on the sterile cloth which is now a safe sterile area for working aseptically.

Step-4

- If necessary or directed, a sterile swab stick is soaked in pus or exudate from the wound. The laboratory sample thus collected is kept separately in a test tube for culture and sensitivity tests.
- A piece of gauze is taken in sponge holding forceps to clean the wound with cleaning solutions.
- In a clean surgical wound, cleaning should be started from centre to periphery and in dirty wound from periphery to the centre.

- The principle of cleaning is to reduce dirty things in the wound but not to contaminate it further.
- In dirty wound, gentle pressure is applied around the wound to see any pus, exudate or blood from unseen pocket. If the bottom of the wound covered with whitish slough, it should be removed by gentle rubbing with gauze or pouring hydrogen peroxide inside. After rubbing, the wound is irrigated with normal saline. The surrounding area is made dry and the wound is covered with Vaseline gauze or any other modern packed dressing (medicated) as and when necessary depending on the type of wound. The oozing wound is covered with absorbent dressing pad.
- In clean surgical wound, dressing is changed without any debridement. Stitches are removed, if the wound is healed and found dry.
- The drain or implant fixation site is also dressed with a separate gauze piece after proper cleaning.
- For holding the dressing covering the wound, adhesive tape or bandage is used.

Step-5

Used gloves and disposable items are disposed of in a clinical waste bag. The reusable items are washed and cleaned and sent for autoclaving.

Step-6

The whole procedure including wound condition should be reported to the physician.

APPLICATION OF PLASTER SLAB

Plaster slab is a rigid immobilization device which supports a part of the circumference of the injured limbs.

Plaster cast, on the other hand, is circumferential immobilizer which is surrounding the whole circumference of the limb.

The plaster slab is prepared by plaster of Paris (POP) bandage which is made of hemi hydrated calcium sulphate. The dry POP bandage, when dipped in water, becomes soft and this soft bandage after a few minutes becomes hard due to chemical changes of its material. The wet plaster can be moulded to any shape because of its softness.

Most of the fractures of limbs are initially immobilized with plaster slab as part of first aid.

Uses

- To immobilize fracture and dislocations of limbs as first aid and also for final treatment in some cases.
- To support hands and feet in tendon injury or tendon surgery.
- To correct the deformity of limbs commonly in club foot treatment.

Materials Required for Application of Plaster Slab

- Plaster of Paris bandage
- Cotton wool
- Bandage roll
- Water in bucket
- Large scissors
- Plaster cutting saw or shears

Technique of Plaster Slab Application

Step-1

- The first step is to confirm the right patient and the right limb where plaster slab will be applied. Plaster application in an incorrect patient or incorrect limb has lot of medicolegal problems.
- The skin condition of the limb should be healthy and free from any wound or ulcer. Blood circulation should be normal and pulsation (radial or posterior tibial or dorsalis pedis) should be checked and noted.

Step-2

- The patient may be in operation table, examination couch, bed, ambulance stretcher or at the accident site. One or two assistants are necessary who can help in holding the limb in correct position.
- The materials required for plaster application are checked and ideally, all the items should be in plaster trolley. The trolley top is used for spreading the plaster roll and a rubber sheet is placed on the top before preparing the slab.

Step-3

- The position of the limb is maintained as instructed by the consultant surgeon.
- The assistant will hold the limb in the selected position.
- Cotton wool is applied to the limb from distal to proximal zone with little stretching force. The cotton layer should be uniform and cover the entire limb. The pressure points of the limbs (joints and bony prominence) are protected well by using proper cotton padding.

Step-4

- Now the length of the slab is measured with the principle that it should cover a joint below and above with exception in few sites.
- Plaster roll is opened from its sealed plastic cover and 6 to 8 layers of the POP bandage of desired length is kept ready for the next step.
- The layer of POP bandage depends on the site and volume of the limb.
- Long leg plaster slab requires more number of the POP roll than that of the below-elbow slab for wrist immobilization.

Step-5

- Two ends of the plaster bandage kept in layers are held with two hands and dipped in water in the bucket till the bubbles cease to come out.

- Then it is taken out of the water kept hanging holding with one hand. The excess water will drop down mechanically.
- The slab is then placed over the trolley top over rubber sheet and rubbed with fingers to remove the air pocket and excess water from the prepared slab.

Step-6

- The slab is now placed on the limb and held in position with the help of cotton bandage roll. Then moulding is done with pressure by the closed fingers. Care should be taken not to create any finger impression over the plaster which might cause plaster sore on the skin.
- It is important to see that the slab will not cross the boundaries of the underlying cotton layers.
- Bandaging should not be too tight or too loose.

- The limb is kept in the desired position until the plaster becomes hard.

Step-7

After the application of the plaster slab, the distal pulse wherever available of the said limb is checked along with colour of the nail bed. Any doubt about pulsation and colour, it should be reported to the physician.

Complication of Plaster Slab

- Itching
- Discomfort
- Allergic skin reaction
- Plaster sore
- Stiffness of the joints
- Wasting of muscles
- Local osteoporosis of bones
- Compartment syndrome with pain and paraesthesia
- Paralysis of nerve
- Limb ischaemia leading to loss of the limb.

CHAPTER 50

Collection, Preservation, and Transport of Samples and Specimens for Pathological Examination

Proper collection, preservation, and transport of surgical specimens are essential for perfect pathological reports. Specimens taken during operation may be a small biopsy or large samples such as entire uterus or kidney.

Collection, preservation, and transport of specimen involve following basic steps:

- Correct identification of the patient.
- Correct identification and confirmation of the specimen by the surgical team.
- Placement of specimen in proper container and preservative.
- Correct labelling of the container.
- Complete pathology requisition slip.
- Transport and handover the specimen to the pathology department.

PROCEDURE OF COLLECTION OF SPECIMEN

- The surgeon must communicate with other team members regarding the specimen.
  - **Type of specimen:** Aerobic or anaerobic, with preservative or without preservative.
  - Types of the diagnostic test to be performed.
  - Anticipated number of specimens.
  - **Requirements of container:** Number and size

- Communications with the pathology department regarding the type of surgical specimen or frozen section.
- Use proper container to protect specimen.
  - The correct size of container to protect specimen.
  - The container should be rigid, unbreakable and non-reactive to fixative.
  - The container should have a tight-fitting cover.

PRESERVATION OF SPECIMEN

- Specimen tissue should be removed very gently to avoid trauma by crushing or tearing of the specimen.
- The specimen should not be allowed to dry out before fixation. If fixation is delayed due to some reasons, specimen should be kept moist with sterile saline or covered by saline-soaked mobs.
- Formalin is the commonest agent used for preservation. The adequate volume of 10% formalin (at least 20:1 ratio) is poured in the container and then gently places the specimen in the container.
- The adequate volume of fixative should be used to cover all the surfaces of specimen.

- The fixation of the large specimen is sometimes difficult. Therefore, they should be rapidly transported to the pathology laboratory for grossing.

TRANSPORTATION OF SPECIMEN

- Before transportation, specimen container should be properly labelled.
- The following information—must be written on the container.
  - Type and site of specimen
  - Patient identification—name and hospital unique ID number
  - Date and time of specimen received
  - Name of surgeon
  - Type of preservative, if used.
- The label should be placed on the side of the container, not on the lid.
- Permanent black or blue ink should be used for labelling.
- Filled up request form should be sent along with the specimen. The following information should be mentioned in the request form.
  - Type and site of sample
  - Patient identifications
  - Relevant clinical history, differential diagnosis, if available, other relevant investigations, if available.
  - Indications of urgency, if any.
- Scrub assistance must take permission from the chief surgeon before hand over the specimen to circulating assistance.
- During the transport, lid of the container should not be opened.
- The specimen is then placed at the collection point of the operation theatre with the complete record in specimen register.
- Fresh/urgent specimens or microbiology samples should also be recorded in register but it must be delivered to respective lab for urgent and prompt action.

- During the transfer of the specimen, chain of custody should be established after recording of specimen in the logbook. Two designated persons are assigned to transfer the specimen in pathology department.
- Pathologist and surgeon should be fixing up the scheduled for pick up/transport of specimens.
- Pathology department should take a leading role in monitoring of transfer of specimen and change of policies, if necessary.

SPECIAL SITUATIONS

Frozen Section

- The operation should be done where facilities for such investigation is available.
- The laboratory should be informed before collection and transport of the specimen.
- It is used mainly for intraoperative diagnosis
- Specimen sent for a frozen section must be fresh without any fixative
- Tissue sent for a frozen section must be processed immediately.
- Therefore, pathologists must be pre-informed and ready for such cases.

Microbiological Test

Aerobic Culture

- Culture specimens should be collected under full aseptic precautions.
- Culture should be obtained by the surgical team by a sterile swab and kept within a sterile test tube.
- Decontaminate the exterior of the culture test tube and transport to microbiology laboratory immediately.

Anaerobic Culture

- Aspirate the fluid by a syringe and recap the tip of the syringe.
- The decontamination of exterior surface is not recommended as it may push the plunger.

- Put the syringe on a sterile container and transport it to microbiology laboratory without any delay.

Foreign Objects of Medicolegal Importance

- All foreign objects of medicolegal importance should be collected, preserved and transported cautiously with an object to preserve all evidence.
- Cut and remove the clothes from the body of the patients with a target to preserve any holes or punctures present on it.
- Clothes should be preserved on the paper bag, not in a plastic bag.

- Wet clothes with blood or body fluids should be placed in a moisture-proof bag to avoid leaking.
- All bags should be labelled for identification.
- Any wound on the surface of the body should be documented in detail.
- The bullet should not be handled with metal instruments because it may cause scratch and distort the evidence.
- The bullet must be cleaned with sterile water to remove blood or tissue. It should be stored in a non-metal container and hand-over to law enforcement officers.

Section VIII

Ethics and Communications

CHAPTER 51

Bioethics

Word ethics is derived from ethos (philosophy). It deals with the right conduct. It helps in distinction between right and wrong at a given time in a given culture with its moral consequence.

Bioethics or medical ethics consists of four basic principles and autonomy, justice, beneficence, veracity and confidentiality. These principles are applicable to all health care providers including operation theatre technologists.

AUTONOMY

Patients have autonomy of thought, intention, and action when making decisions regarding treatment for their illness. Autonomy of patients means they have right to choose or refuse their treatment.

BENEFICENCE

Beneficence means actions that promote the well-beings of others. In the medical profession, treatment modality should be chosen to serve best interests of patients and their families.

The job of health care providers is to do 'good' for the patient. Their goal should be to preserve life, restore health and relieve suffering.

NON-MALEFICENCE

Means "first do no harm". It is more important "not to harm patients than to do good". Every treatment modality carries certain risks and it is important to calculate the risk-benefit ratio. It is the job of health care providers to explain all possible side effects or complications of proposed treatment modality. Competency of health care provider should be analyzed to prevent undue risk to the patients due to inadequate experience or training.

VERACITY

Means 'truth-telling', it is the duty of health care provider to discuss with patients about their illness in details. There should be full and honest disclosure about entire course and possible outcome of disease.

CONFIDENTIALITY

During the course of treatment, many personal matters of the patient may be revealed to the health care provider. It is the job of the health care provider to maintain the confidentiality of all personnel, medical or treatment information. It should not be disclosed except for legal reasons.

JUSTICE AND SOCIAL RESPONSIBILITY

Actions of health care providers should be transparent. They must be fair to all patients and there should not be any discrimination on the basis of age, sex, religion, race, position or rank.

All doctors, nurses, technologists, and other hospital staff must be aware of all ethical issues related to patient care and should strictly follow the guideline to avoid litigations. In operation theatre, some other points should also be considered because patient may be under general anaesthesia or under the influence of sedatives or narcotics.

ETHICAL ISSUES IN THE OPERATION THEATRE

- **Dress:** Before the transfer of the patient to operation theatre, sterile dress is offered for change.
  - The dress should provide adequate cover according to local standards (religion).
  - The dress should provide adequate local (selective) exposure.
  - The dress should allow quick and practical wide exposure in emergency situations.
  - The dress should look descent.
- **People gathering and traffic:**
  - Often too many people in the corridors, receiving area and operation theatre, cause inconvenience to patients and staff. Ensure selective people entry in the operation theatre, in the ward. Limit the number of personnel in the operation room during preparation and surgery especially for female patients.
  - Try and ensure not to carry out any procedures during visiting hours.
  - In a medical college, undergraduate students would always be present. Ensure a good learning environment for the students and a comfortable environment for the patient. Check on the patient once in a while, to see for discomfort. Try to ensure that other patients are not getting disturbed.
- **Exposure of body:**
  - In the case of female patients, always work in presence of a female nurse.
  - Exposure of body parts is often necessary, depending on the procedure. Hence exposure is to be limited to parts needed only.
  - Exposure of the body of the patient is to be done in the presence of the limited number of people.
  - Exposure of the body of the patient is to be done for the shortest period of time.
  - Preserve patients' dignity during all phases of transportation.
  - Patient examination, if needed, should be inside the operating room with privacy and limited exposure.
- **Noise:**
  - Patients coming to operation theatre are worried. They would need privacy, silence, and reassurance.
  - Noise should be kept to a minimum.
- **Comments and behaviour:**
  - Avoid jokes and laughing:
    - Loudly
    - In front of patients
    - In a language not known to them
    - Before anaesthesia
    - During procedure with local/spinal anaesthesia.
  - Avoid comments and remarks on the patient:
    - Related to disease
    - Body shape or weight
    - Behaviour.
  - Avoid using phones for reasons other than important receiving or making calls.
  - Keep the instrument tray properly covered, maintaining sterility. Ensure that the patient is not able to see the instruments before anaesthesia. It would increase their stress.

- **Honesty:**
  - Patients often ask who performed surgery. While answering keep in mind:
    - Clarify the concept of teamwork.
    - Assure about quality.
    - Emphasize on supervision by the consultant/senior staff.
    - Assure that teaching/training does not reduce standards
  - Tell the truth regarding:
    - What went wrong,
    - Complications, or
    - Unexpected incidence should be discussed in details by team leader only. Comments by other team members may create confusion and unnecessary dissatisfaction.
  - The operation theatre technologist, because of his position and presence inside the operation theatre will come to know about various aspects of the patient's life and status. He/she should always keep in mind that whatever was learned inside must be kept inside. No details of the patient can be divulged to a third person. Health care personal and patient confidentiality must never be disclosed, except:
    - In a court of law under orders of the presiding judge,
    - In case of notifiable diseases,
    - In circumstances where there is a serious and identified risk to a specific person and/or community.

INFORMED CONSENT

- A person must be fully informed about the treatment options, potential risks, and benefits of their choice of treatment.
- Similarly patient has the right to refuse the treatment. Potential risks and benefits related to treatment refusal should also be explained. This is called informed refusal.
- Adult patients are eligible to give consent for treatment.
- When patients are incapacitated or not in a position to take the decision for himself or herself, their next of kin make decisions for them.
- Should not be taken in the operating room.

CHAPTER 52

Attitude and Communications

Communication is an important component in the health care field. Employees in hospitals, nursing homes, and other medical settings need to communicate regularly with patients and residents about medical procedures, daily care tasks, and the patient's overall health. **Communication can be defined as the ability to convey or share ideas and feelings effectively**. Effective health care personnel–patient communication can improve quality of care, clinical outcomes, and health care personnel–patient relationship that enhances patient satisfaction.

The different types of communications are:

- Verbal communication
  - Formal communication
  - Informal communication
- Non-verbal communication
- Written communication

VERBAL COMMUNICATION

Verbal communication can also be called oral communication. In very simple terms, any communication that happens orally between people is known as verbal communication.

The objective of such communications is to ensure that people understand whatever you want to convey. They meet with many patients, with different problems in the course of their treatment. Each patient is different in terms of their understanding and talking skills. Thus, operation theatre technologists need to have excellent verbal communication skills.

In a hospital setting, two types of verbal communication are present—formal and informal verbal communication.

Formal Communication

Formal communication can be very rigid, leaving little or no room for feedback or deviation. Health care workers use formal communication when explaining the disease, treatment protocol, explaining a procedure and hospital policies to patients and their families.

Informal Communication

Informal communication includes enquiring about other aspects of the patients' life which are not directly related to their disease. Informal communications with patients may include discussions about their hobbies, interests, favourite singer or author. Informal verbal communication is used mostly to make the patient feel comfortable and reduce the stress-related to a hospital visit.

NON-VERBAL COMMUNICATION

Non-verbal communication is the body language of the health care personnel. It is not said by the person but includes the gestures, the way the operation theatre technologist touches the patient, how he greets the patient.

Non-verbal communication is silent but at times it is stronger than verbal communication. A panicked operation theatre technologist in the operation theatre, in a non-ironed uniform, without a reassuring smile and a cold hand will definitely increase the fear of the patient.

WRITTEN COMMUNICATION

It is, in reality, a type of formal communication. It is often found in hospital policies and documents. It is mostly used to put a definite directive in writing for the patient. The importance of written communication are:

* To make sure that the care and treatment can continue to be given safely no matter which staff is on duty, 24 hours a day, seven days a week.
* To record the care that has been given to the patient.
* To make sure there is an accurate record to be used as 'evidence' when there is a complaint from a patient about the care they have received.
* To obtain written consent from the patient in presence of their relatives as witness for their treatment, different procedures including operations.

Operation theatre technicians along with the operation theatre nurses are the first group of people who come in contact with the patients in the operation theatre. The basic communication skills required for an operation theatre technician can be tabulated as follows:

Towards the Patient

* **Greet the patient with a soothing smile:**
  - Enquire and confirm the name and age of the patient with respect and dignity and make them feel important. Address them by the first name on subsequent visits give a sense of being taken care of.
  - In the case of a planned operation, a gentle"Good morning, how are you feeling today? How was your sleep last night?" can be a good stress reliever for the patient.
* **Present with a calm attitude:**
  - Visiting a hospital as a patient is never an easy experience. Patients are fearful, apprehensive about the future.
  - The calmness in the behaviour of the health care personnel will assure and calm down the patient.
  - The communication with the patients in a calm assuring voice with a smiling face makes them feel assured and secure.
  - Talking about funny incidents, sharing a decent joke and talking about things the patient is interested in, makes the patient relaxed.
* **Avoid to use the medical term as much as possible and to communicate in patient's own language:**
  - Try to avoid technical terms as much as possible. Explain patients' physical condition and treatment protocol in common language which layman can understand easily.
  - It increases compliance and adaptability of the patient to the hospital environment.
  - For example, during discharge, if a patient is asked "to monitor water intake and output 12 hourly", it may be difficult for patient to follow instructions. It may be easy to understand, if they are instructed to write down how much they drink and how many times they urinate every 2 hours, would give a better idea about their intake and output.
* **Assure and reassure the patient regarding the operation:**
  - It is without any doubt that a patient would be extremely apprehensive about

an operation. It is preferable to explain the sequence of events that will occur during the perioperative stay.

– Talking about the past patients who benefitted from a similar procedure/s helps the patient to relax.

– Emphasizing the professionalism of the surgical team and their intent towards the benefit of the patient gives them a lot of confidence.

- **Treat every patient with empathy** (the ability to understand and share the feelings of another):

  – It is not necessary for every health care professional to go through the same experience, but trying to make the patients feel that their fear, concern, apprehensions are understandable, creates a soothing effect on the patients' psychology and gives the necessary confidence to face the situation.

  – For example, if a mother with small child at home is admitted at hospital for some illnesses, and if health care provider expresses that he can understand the difficulties of staying in hospital without child. If he assures that everything will be fine and she will be discharged soon" may boost up the mood of the patient.

- **Touch the patient with dignity and respect, with due permission:**

  – In the ward and the operation theatre, the health care personnel will have to touch the patient for examination, measuring blood pressure, giving an injection, etc.

  – Take permission and explain the technique. This prevents lot of future problems and misunderstandings.

  – It is advisable to wash the hand before and after touching the patient to avoid the spread of infection.

  – In cold weather, touching the patient with cold hands will definitely irritate him/her. Making their own hands warm by rubbing will make the patient comfortable when touched for examination.

  – During procedures where the patient is awake and conscious, like during administration spinal or epidural anaesthesia, reassurance and gentle touch on the hand or shoulders of the patient eases the apprehension.

- **Give the patient full attention. Never seem rushed or frustrated with the patient:**

  – Patients are generally very anxious before any procedure.

  – Postoperative patients may talk incoherently under the influence of anaesthetic drugs. The operation theatre technologist is expected to present with a calm attitude, without any frustration of answering the same question repeatedly.

  – Checking the time repeatedly or the mobile phone repeatedly gives the patient an impression of inattentiveness.

  – An apathetic look of the technical persons in the theatre is not liked by the patient.

As a Member of the Surgical Team

The operation theatre technician plays a very important role in the operation theatre team. They must understand and obey the instruction given by the surgeon and/or nursing staff. Excellent communication skill supported by his technical skill is essential to carry out entire procedure smoothly. The specific communication skills required are:

- **Understand and respond proactively** to the need of an operating surgeon.

  – Operation theatre technologists must know the basic steps of operation and the type of instruments required.

  – Knowing these facts ensures an easier and smoother operation.

  – Close monitoring of the procedure and hand over the instruments as per the necessity helps to save a lot of time.

- **Cool tempered with emotional and physical stamina:**
  - Operation theatre technologist should not leave the operation theatre until the patient is recovered from anaesthesia and shifted to the recovery room.
  - Vital parameters must be recorded and reported to the on-duty nurse during handover process of the patient at the post-anaesthesia care unit.
  - It is necessary for the person to be cool-tempered to face any query from the patient's relatives and friends. It is desirable to convey the message that surgeon and anaesthesiologist will meet the relatives and explain everything related to patients.

- **Behave as a team member with excellent communication skills:**
  - Operation theatre is a very tense place, with stress levels very high. In this situation, everyone is dependent on the performance of the previous person to complete their work effectively.
  - This requires the ability to work as a team. Passing information from the surgical team to the relatives of the patient can be extremely crucial during the operation.
  - Good communication skill of the person helps to pass the information such as requirement of more blood, drugs or implants due to some unusual condition occurred during surgery.
  - It requires the person to be calm, composed and dignified during an interaction.

- **Good understanding of patient safety and precautions:**
  - The well-being of the patient is of paramount importance in the operation theatre.
  - So understanding the measures for patient safety and the necessary precautions to maintain patient safety ensures the well-being of the patient.

- **Understanding hierarchy and follow the guideline of the hospital:**
  - As the operation theatre is a closed, extremely confidential space, so the operation theatre technologist must assure that nothing goes out.
  - There is only one designated spokes-person for that matter. The patient is always admitted under the care of a doctor, and the doctor usually communicates and counsels the patient and relatives during preoperative period.
  - So it is imperative and an unwritten rule that information from the operation theatre should be passed only by concerned doctors or any person designated by them.

Index